SEAS OF YELLOW

SEAS OF YELLOW

BECOMING FRIENDS WITH MY MENTAL HEALTH

LEVI SANTHA

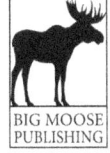

BIG MOOSE
PUBLISHING

©2024 Levi Santha. All rights reserved.
Published by: Big Moose Publishing
PO Box 127 Site 601 RR#6 Saskatoon, SK CANADA S7K 3J9
www.bigmoosepublishing.com

This book is a truthful recollection of actual events in the author's life. This book represents the personal views and opinions of the author and does not necessarily reflect the positions or opinions of any organization, institution, or individual with which the author is affiliated. The content presented herein is based on the author's perspective and interpretation of the subject matter. Neither the publisher nor any associated parties shall be held responsible for any consequences arising from the opinions or interpretations expressed within this book.

Some names have been changed in order to protect the identity of those mentioned in the book. Others have been kept true, and those individuals have granted permission for their names to be used.

Printed in Canada.

ISBN: 978-1-989840-70-2 (sc)
ISBN: 978-1-989840-71-9(e)
Big Moose Publishing 03/24

DEDICATION

For my sons, Milo and Denny.
In a world that can be cruel, be kind. In a world that can be
distant, be personal. In a world that can be fictional, be you.
You are going to accomplish incredible feats.
Love, Papa.

CONTENTS

PROLOGUE

I've always loved stories. The movement of a character waltzing through both trial and tribulation provides me with context as to who they become at the final page or scene. There is something beautiful about the contrast between their previous and post self that oftentimes illustrates the candid realities of their experiences.

This book is my story, so far. It may not appear as "state-of-the-art" or revolutionary like those seen in Hollywood blockbuster flicks. In those cases, the protagonist manages to retain a sense of composure about themselves as the war erupts around them. Alongside the immense challenges and prejudice, they rebound back from an emotional episode and charge up and over the line of the trench defiantly. My story has not always benefited from the romantic ideals that exist in the hearts of those looking to be entertained.

Perhaps the purpose of this text is to achieve some sort of therapeutic liberation. That I am not quite sure of just yet. Nonetheless, I have felt an indescribable desire to put my thoughts to paper. With hope, maybe you can relate to some of my thoughts. Perhaps you may sense comfort in knowing that there are other people in the world who are attempting to find peace with themselves, all the while being reminded of their delicate past.

I want to personally thank you for allowing this overanalyzing, hypercritical mind to share in transparency.

CHAPTER ONE

SEAS OF YELLOW

As the light bounced off of the crops of canola and into the windows of the SUV, I couldn't help but notice that I was entranced in the brief moment of peace and serenity. This feeling consumed the utmost of my attention. Each individual stem within the field budded with a pastel of yellows and ambers that remained delightful to the eye. Naturally, the intense contrast of the expanse was heightened due to the atmosphere of blue that reigned overtop it. When one looked into the distance, it was difficult to tell if the exposure would eventually be tamed by an approaching cloud front or prairie storm.

It was August. During the summer period, driving through mid-southern Saskatchewan was considered an "eye-chore" for the typical local. Sparks of spontaneity, which were few and far between, would consist of passing motorcades of semis hauling freight to God knows where. The clashing of opposing wind fronts would not only move the vehicle itself, but would send a deafening leer into one's ears, causing momentary panic. Perchance, the vehicle one was riding in would pass the remnants of an animal carcass slumped on the shoulder of the asphalt. Of course, not much organic material would be left thanks to the opportunistic nature of the crows and coyotes. But despite the tedium, August was special. The once barren landscapes would suddenly burst with life. Sprouts of green would begin to poke up from within the soil, and with a faint touch of Mother Nature's care, seas of yellow would spout forth in spectacular fashion.

This re-emergence of life had oftentimes felt melancholic to me. With the arrival of summer crops, it signalled that my vacation time away from school and other formal responsibilities was fleeting. Sitting introspectively in my seat, I attempted to tune out the chaos that was exploding amongst my other familial passengers. The feeling of being confined to such a small area, restricted by the noose of a seatbelt, left me starving for what existed outside the windowpane. The moments to admire the scenery were waning. I may not have realized it at the time, but my mind was already beginning to fortify itself for an unknown, yet expected assault of the senses. It was routine. It was recognizable.

Although I had been born in "The City of Bridges" (Saskatoon), I was quick to refer to the areas of Lake Diefenbaker as my true home. Reason for such a belief was thanks to my parents, whom made the intentional decision to invest in the inherited family cottage when time arose. This sanctuary was located in the sleepy little villa of Mistusinne.

For my two younger brothers and I, the opportunities presented for holistic personal growth at Mistusinne were like that of an untapped goldmine. Tidbits of unrefined ore took form in the shape of various activities. One could partake in unsupervised walks down the water's shoreline. One could discover the hives of protective yellow jackets, taunting the idea of having a stone thrown at them. One could brave the elements of the nearby slough and catch frogs by the bucketful. It was paradise.

But for what it had in plenty, Mistusinne lacked in practicality. The village has, and continues to, lack modern amenities such as village-wide sewage irrigation, local grocery options, and policing. It's as if its founders in 1980 decided that the community would benefit from a more traditional way of life that reflected both rural neighbourly interactions and isolated pockets of independence. For example, if one was in dire need of a particular resource, such as a gallon of milk or roll of toilet paper, their best bet would be to take a walk of shame to the house next door and request for it humbly. In most cases, such a request was not intrusive at all. This was of course reflective of the village's "reciprocity act" that went unofficial, yet appeared strangely, collectively understood. Should there be no luck in pandering to the folks nearby, one would have to take the short drive to the nearby town of Elbow or Tugaske. Albeit, purchasing foodstuffs from the independent grocer was the equivalent of purchasing fruit in the northern regions of the Northwest Territories. It was just as expensive as it was selective.

Medical emergencies would prove to be a unique kind of predicament, as local paramedics would have to conduct lengthy patient transfers to better equipped institutions located in places such as Saskatoon or Moose Jaw. For the notable elderly population at Mistusinne, it seemed high risk to choose such a place for retirement. But perhaps they had already made the mental trade off of choosing to perish in a remote, dreamy place than that of an overcrowded old-folks home. There was no fear of forced interaction, no fear of consuming subpar food, and there was definitely no fear of picky schedules to adhere to. The thought was tantalizing, and I would have to return to it the year I turned 65. Nonetheless, one would consider themselves fortunate if a medical evacuation were never to happen prior to late adulthood.

While some may have interpreted Mistusinne as purgatory, others (like myself) saw it as a place of solace. Upon pulling into the makeshift dirt driveway of the cabin, there was a noticeable feeling as if time had not passed since the visitor's last interaction. The (for lack of a better term) cute, little shack would appear untouched. It served as an architectural time capsule of sorts. Undoubtedly, its physical impression left much to be desired. The wood monument had been subjected to numerous facial afflictions over the years, caused by the many weather systems colliding with one another above the nearby lake reservoir. It was common for hail stones the size of golf balls to rain down on the area, causing widespread property damage and dread. All that would remain afterwards was dented vehicles, damaged homes, and an overwhelming ocean of melting ice. Paint chips on the cabin had cracked and fallen to the base of the structure, leaving a metaphorical display of crows-feet and aging on the building's complexion.

Inside, the building smelled of stale winter air, partially viewed VHS tapes, and expired sunscreen lotion. I had always commented on how if a company had managed to capture such a musk within a candle, they would ensure at least one repeat customer. Weird sounding, rightly so, but I imagine that others have their own version of this strange affinity to scents. Afterwards, I would instinctively make my way to my room, a tiny area located at the north-end side of the cabin, and haphazardly throw my packed bag onto the mattress as a physical gesture of claiming the space. I had been fortunate after all to be the eldest of three siblings. I was privileged with having a room all to myself. The irony in this would later be realized when I grew tall enough that my feet would dangle off of the end of the bed as I slept, but it beat having to share the room with another person.

On the other hand, my brothers were cohabiting a room across the hall. However, the term "room" perhaps does not accurately define the dimensions of this space. It resembled the size of a walk-in closet. From my place of solitude, I could often hear an argument ensue across the hall. The cause? Who laid claim to the top bunk of the double-decker bunkbed! Thankfully, these confrontations were often short and settled themselves through empty threats and one's disappointment in acquiring the lower confine. Eventually, the person who "won" the top bunk would later realize that the earlier victory was but an unfortunate misconception. Morning would start off fairly cool and pleasant, temperature wise. But as the day progressed, heat would enter through the front door and windows and roast all within the house like food in a pressure cooker. In this case, it paid off for my youngest brother to have lost to seniority and be sanctioned to the bottom bunk.

I was finally home. I would be for the next several days and weeks. My first mission to accomplish was to forget everything there was about Saskatoon and anyone that pertained to it. I wouldn't be able to see any evidence of it, so it may as well have never existed. All that was left of it was memories and the smell of laundry detergent in the clean clothes that were brought with. That would soon disappear.

The freedom that this villa provided me with was picturesque, comparable to what one would expect from a childhood utopia like Mark Twain's Huckleberry Finn. One aspect of freedom looked like building forts out of the tree debris in the most remote areas of the village. This was often away from the eyes and ears of adults. The only major downfall to this activity were the bloodsucking ticks that managed to latch onto the bare skin of my legs as I waded through overgrown patches of grass. Their movement is virtually unrecognizable, and their grip is sure to cause alarm when they don't come off of the body with a light tug. Such a realization of these horrible parasites is why ticks continue to haunt me to this day.

Some days, I saw myself pacing the lakefront, scrutinizing every piece of rock and sediment on the beach. The goal was to find some form of ancient treasure, whether that be eye-catching pyrite (Fool's Gold), or better yet, archaeological remains. In fact, well before European settlement of the region, Lake Diefenbaker had been home to a prospering and diverse plains-Indigenous population. These peoples had followed the hordes of bison, making nomadic lifestyle a staple of their practices. They worshipped the Creator who had provided in abundance to them the food, water, and community that was necessary for cultural survival. Indeed, the region was home to many sacred locations where reverence was a common practice. One such location was noted on the southern slope of the valley which preceded the eventual flooding of the district at the hands of the Gardiner Dam. On the slope sat an enormous venerated stone. It was routinely worshipped by the Cree/Nehiyaw people, who coined the stone in their native tongue "Mistaseni", meaning "Big Rock". It was fitting for the future village to be named after such an honoured material.

My efforts in searching for the presence of this intriguing people did not go unrewarded. Within a span of two years, when I was roughly 13-15 years old, I was able to find two stone arrowheads. Each object had been laying prone in the sand and was unique in composition and size. I tend to credit these archaeological discoveries as the inspiration for my eventual career choice as a history teacher. It has also made me aware that their finding had instilled in me the desire to learn more about those that lived before us. These objects made me feel as though I was able to look at Mistusinne for the past that it was.

Other days, the only significant adventure I would have was related to fishing. After loading up a plastic bucket with whatever worn-down fishing rod, spoons, jigs, and net that I could find in the cottage garage, I would bike down to the local boat launch. From there I would scale down the rocky encampment of the bluff, rip off my sandals when I reached the beach, and wade knee-to-waist deep in the brisk evening water. Cast after cast I was able to bask in the euphoric moments of peace. I would stand still, so not to scare the fish away, and revel in the knowledge that Saskatchewan truly was the "Land of Living Skies". Reflecting off of the crystalline waters of the lake were shades of pink, orange, and even reds resembling the sharp tones of ochre. The bail of the rod would be flipped, my pointer finger would grip the fishing line, and subsequently was cast out twenty feet until I heard a soft "plop!". With a "click!", the reel would be functional for retrieving the cast, and the cyclical, hypnotic process would continue. These images were breathtaking, to say the least.

Yet despite the amount of sovereignty felt throughout these experiences, I could always feel my subconscious plucking me back into a place of mental insecurity. In the back of my mind, flashes (scenes even) controlled my attention like an insect unable to distract itself from a lightbulb. I could hear the disembodied cries of people fighting and screaming at one another. I was typically unable to identify one specific instance or distraction that could pierce my perception of reality. It would keep me in a state where I was unable to live consciously in the moment. A sense of tenseness would lock my chest into place, making it difficult to feel like I could breathe efficiently. Worst of all, it was maddening to slip into a state of paranoia.

Why was it, in moments such as these, that finding a place of mental harbouring was not possible? How do I stay afloat in this tossing ocean that is life? As the fishing rod in my hands was slowly wound in, the nip of a walleye at the end of the line would pull me away from these poisonous thoughts. My younger self would not have been able to recognize what was happening. My mind was in a battle. At some point, I had to go back home. If only I could have been able to tell him what I know now. I would tell him that trauma performs in perplexing ways.

"The strongest oak of the forest is not the one that is protected from the storm and hidden from the sun. It's the one that stands in the open where it is compelled to struggle for its existence against the winds and rains and the scorching suns."

– Napoleon Hill

CHAPTER TWO

THREE HOMES, MANY REALITIES

As mentioned before, Saskatoon was where I was born and raised. It's mid-central geography within the province allowed for a devious combination of seasons ranging from balmy summer days to blisteringly frigid winter nights. Despite the fragility of weather constants, the "Paris of the Prairies" title given to the city certainly appears earned after brief inspection. When one walks the trails of the South Saskatchewan River (which happens to wind its way right through the centre of the city), it is impossible to not be entertained by the flurry of natural energy that exists. From time to time, despite its exponential civil and industrial growth, Saskatoon has been able to entertain its human residents by reminding them that nature is still around. Animals such as coyotes, deer, and even moose manage to infiltrate city limits and make their way into the suburban neighbourhoods, albeit with understandable distress and confusion. I wonder if their predicaments are made even more confusing because of their primal knowledge of what this place had been like before people arrived?

What I neglected to mention at first was that although I was born at the Royal University Hospital in 1996, my parents at the time had been living in a remote town in the far north region of the province. From the knowledge that I was given growing up, my mother (Tracy) and father (Jason) had moved upwards to the small rural community of La Loche due to a variety of personal circumstances. First, and assumedly, Mom had been faced with several relational issues with her own parents which incited the need for distance. Such explanations that we children had been told seemed valid. We were simply too young to understand how to achieve effective solutions to quell social tensions. Secondly, the move had made more sense knowing that two of my father's siblings (my eldest aunt and uncle) had been working in the area previous to their arrival. So, Dad joined his brother in running a confectionary store that doubled as a video game arcade. I grew up listening to countless stories of this haven. My father recounted the fun-spirited atmosphere that flooded the building, which included the ability for one to consume any deep fried food item they wanted. If one wanted to try their luck at the joystick of a Mortal Combat machine, they could simply unlock the coin slots to the system and recycle quarters at a lawless expense. I can imagine scenes of Dad, working behind the opening of a kitchen window, belting out lyrics to *The Tragically Hip's* "New Orleans Is Sinking", and dunking a vat of french fries into the depths of a deep fryer. It must have felt surprisingly calm to know that the only task at hand was to pump food out for solitary orders and to wipe down game controls at the end of a shift. But despite the overall charm that these stories displayed, there was an undermining reality that had often been left out.

La Loche is a town predominantly made up by a Dene and Cree Indigenous population. My parents, faced with the obvious fact that they were one of the few visible minorities in town, elicited mixed reviews from the locals because of their notable (different) presence. However, it is integral to note that much of the negative interaction between my folks and the community stems from a larger, more significant origin. That origin being colonial history. It is understandable, to a degree, that skepticism would fester between both parties. These concerns, doubled with the added challenge that many families were living in or below the poverty line, meant that terrible things would happen from time to time. The lesser, but still intimidating, act of taunting and physical aggression had continued to strike an uncomfortable level of fear into my parents. For instance, the reactionary decision to purchase a fully-trained, retired police dog named "Sas" (Dene for "Bear") seemed like a strategic choice. Sas was a German Shepard, and was familiar with defensive takedown procedures for when strangers came too close to one's family. Cue the visuals of a mouth-full of teeth and startling lunges.

Matters would take a turn for the worse when, on a series of occasions, someone would break into the store, set off the alarms, and cause chaos in the dark of the night. Because our living quarters were attached to an offset portion of the confectionary, the burglary felt intrusive of personal space and safety. Although I was never told of the specifics, I can imagine that a Louisville Slugger napped from within the corner of a door-space, waiting for its time to shine! Needless to say, after a series of unsettling events, Mom and Dad agreed that staying in La Loche to raise a family would prove to be an unfit decision.

There was only one major issue with this decision: money. Mom and Dad had lived frugally, as a result of working simple jobs with low pay rates. To move meant that a multitude of financial factors were to be considered. This included securing affordable transportation for the ride down to urban civilization, and it also meant that they had to lock down living arrangements. To cover the cost of newborn diapers and general groceries like canned soups and frozen dinners, payments would be made on a VISA Card. Thus began the steep and slippery descent into debt that was felt (and vocalized) by my parents in the years to come. Was it survival or was it simplicity? I'm not quite sure. Regardless, the reverberations of my Dad's voice saying "Never get a credit card" continue to play in my head as I sit here and write. Maybe the answer is all in the wording.

As a result of this lifestyle development, Mom and Dad were to make the difficult decision to move back to Saskatoon and live with her parents, my Grandma and Grandpa (*Oma* and *Opa* as I call them to this day). It comes as no surprise that such a resolve was required in order to stay afloat. Traditionalists by nature, my grandparents apply their conservative Christian Reformed ideals to their lives' circumstances like the reverent Protestants they are. Life was to be interpreted like a chess match. Sure, there were elements of sacrifice involved in maintaining some semblance of order, but moves were to be made with calculated precision. Moves were especially to be made one at a time. The short, feisty Dutch couple also benefitted from the ability to switch between the English and Dutch language, so to covertly communicate their responses to one another. As for my parents, there is no doubt that this vacancy appeared more like a binding contract. They must have felt some form of internal strife and guilt knowing that they had caved on their previous reasonings for leaving Saskatoon, especially as they were coming to terms with the fact that they had lost their personal battle to stay away.

It was my Opa, the stout jovial man equipped with a greying moustache, who managed to get my father a job in the back warehouse of a local industrial piping company. The job itself was as a pipe technician. It wasn't pretty, and it consisted mainly of repetitional cycles of cutting, welding, and shipping PVC material day in and day out. If one could fortify their mental patience, perhaps the routine could be softened with a bi-weekly paycheque that was superior to a task that garnered minimum wage. Regardless of the quality of work, Dad was able to slowly work himself up into a position of authority. Of course, this was assisted with the presence of a surly father-in-law whom was no stranger to speaking his mind when it came to political or workplace incidents. A beneficial ally Opa was, to be sure! From the warehouse, Dad moved into the sales office. This work was quite the contrast from technician work, as it traded the tools of a fusion machine for a desktop computer and wired telephone. And while I hadn't seen my Dad's talents in person, I had known that he was becoming quite skilled in the trade. The steady flow of a salary had allowed our family to move out of my grandparents' dwelling and into a new home of our very own. Never before had our standards of living improved to such a degree! The relief that my Oma and Opa must have felt becoming empty-nesters for the second time in their lives…

The house that my parents purchased happened to be on 11th Street. To my uninformed and childish perception, it was a wonderful and cozy little abode. Light blue paint veneered across its four exterior walls, a surprisingly large backyard was guarded by 7 foot tall fence board, and there was a room for every person to make petition to. Bountiful. By this point I was two years old, was beginning to grow into my tiny body, and was exploring the world around me. I also was not doing it alone. My mother had become pregnant while living at my grandparents, and subsequently gave birth to another son shortly after moving into the blue house. They named him Liam. He was a spunky baby, and was quick to do things that would want my parents to both belt out in laughter and rip the hair out of their skulls. My memory recalls a floor rug having baby powder professionally imbued with the stuff.

With two bedrooms located in the upstairs segment of the house, it meant that both Liam and I were to share a room that was the size of a closet. Although it wasn't, it felt smaller than the bunkbed room at the cabin. That feeling could be blamed on the presence of various cupboards and dressers that had been jammed in alongside the assortment of children's toys. For $30,000, the investment of the fixer-upper property had already seemed to be making its mark. Our days were spent sprinting from the back of the house to the top of a rickety play structure (whose emergence was unknown to me). Certain days would have us cling to the height of the structure and call out to the neighbour kids across the street to inquire on whether or not they could play. Other days, I would sit in the dingy, cold, and frankly dirty basement and watch cartoons on the smallest Panasonic television that one could imagine.

One fond memory sticks out the most, amongst the others. For my fifth birthday, Mom decided to theme a party for me around one of my favourite things: dinosaurs. My mother, a naturally gifted artist and creative, hand drew and crafted various saurian related visuals and placed them around the property. Additionally, my father filled up balloons with water and allowed the invitees to go berserk for a short period of time. To finish off the day, we sat around the living room table and ate a small, pre-assembled Safeway cake. Each guest was sent off with a dinosaur themed gift bag, for good measure, by the end of the event. Everything was perfect. I know now to interpret and reflect upon this memory with great admiration and respect for my Mom and Dad, for it had created a moment in time for me that was invaluable without the need to focus on spending money. Such a focus on monetary value would become increasingly apparent in our future years.

Moving day may stand out as one of the worst days in my entire life. I had just turned eight-years-old, and the once large home had seemingly shrunk. At six years of age, my family had welcomed yet another child into the world. You guessed it, another boy. With respect to the compact blue house, something had to give. In order to make living accommodations functional, I was moved from the now three-person communal bedroom to one in the basement. It was previously used as a storage room and was startlingly cold. Even this act of movement could not subdue my parents' ever-growing desire to move into a home that was more practical for a family of five. I can't and don't blame them for thinking so.

There were other factors that led to this decision. Some were so apparent that it was difficult to ignore them. For starters, the basement had a faulty drainage system. On occasion, as laundry was being done, water of questionable roots would rise up from a pipe in the middle of the room, slide across the tiling, and seep into the nearby carpet. The aftermath left a peculiar scent, even after Pine-Sol had been used to scrub the space from floor to ceiling. Another motive for the move had to be the neighbourhood itself. Many of my memories associated with moving into that basement room include the sounds of police sirens, particularly at night. Across the street was an independent grocer called T*he Lew Brothers*. Run by two brothers of the same last name, the store served as a quick option to purchase last minute items needed for breakfast, lunch, and dinner. The two Mr. Lew's were incredibly generous men. From time to time, Dad would walk us boys across the jostling street to buy some groceries. Upon placing the items on the conveyor belt, the brothers would forcibly convince him to let each of us kids find a snack and rentable VHS film to take home, free of charge. They did so with smiles on their faces and genuine love for the reactions that we would offer them in return.

I could not imagine how these men dealt with the challenges

that they were given. Their store was suspect to many a break-in. Property was often stolen and vandalized. One night, after a homeless man had broken into the change dispenser of a nearby payphone, he began shouting vulgar threats to the sky, pacing back and forth in front of the store's entrance in an erratic manner. Similar to my parent's home in La Loche, the store also doubled as the Lew brothers' home. It was my folks that had called the police to come and mitigate the situation. I remember the faint distress in my mother's tone as she questioned how long we could all live with this nearby reality. The spasming patterns of red and blue permeated through the blinds of our home and etched a lasting impression in my youthful mind.

Yet another memory that clearly reprises itself to me from time to time happens to be on a night where I had just lied down to go to bed. After pulling my Scooby-Doo blanket overtop of my head, I had been startled by an unknown noise. A light knocking sound could be heard coming from the basement window that overlooked my bedroom. Confused, and wondering if my Dad had gone outside to play a prank on me, I lifted the covers and stood on the top of my mattress to investigate the cause of the sound. Upon pulling back the curtains, the clear face of a man with bulging eyes and a terrifying smile stared back at me. I screamed. I had woken up both of my siblings in the process as I galloped up the stairs, pleading for my parents to provide some sort of context for what had just happened. After some convincing, Dad agreed to investigate the perimeter of the house, but claimed to have never found or seen anything out of the ordinary. I pleaded with him to phone my neighbour friend's father across the street to see if it was him who had initiated the deed. Dad's response sent a shiver down my spine. He was out of town on a business trip. To this day, I am unsure whether my own father was messing with me, or if in reality some intoxicated stranger really had been watching me through the window.

Despite all of its flaws, that home holds a lot of sentiment to me. Many of my formative years were spent there. Some of these times included those in which I attended pre-school, made my very first non-relative friends, and grew to become interested in certain topics and extracurricular activities that would guide me into becoming the person that I am today. My parents had hired a realtor to sell the home. Needless to say, I hated her. It is not that I hated her as a person for her qualities, because I am sure she was a lovely woman. I just hated what she was doing, which was selling something that provided me so much happiness. The final day of our ownership of that home was one that I will never forget. The realtor provided us her congratulations, gave each of us kids a wide smile and gentle wave, and then bid us farewell. All of the months that were spent upgrading, improving the aesthetic, and showcasing our home were officially over. It was time to move on. I took one final, solemn walk through the empty house and mourned for what was. There was nothing that I could logically do to hold on to this place any longer.

A huge undertaking was presented to us when my parents bought a house on the opposite side of the river. Located in Saskatoon's *Avalon* neighbourhood, the house that they purchased was of a much larger scale compared to the tiny blue home that sat on 11th Street. It was a bungalow, straight from the 1950's, and had been furnished with decor and modifications to match the time era it had come from. It was a mansion to a child's eyes. Seeing as we moved around the fall/winter season, us children immediately asserted dominance over various sections of the front lawn to use as bases for snow forts. Inside, a moderately sized living area, bathroom, and several bedrooms were sprawled across the upper level. That left a laundry room, small living area, and a single bedroom locked to the basement. It was only natural for me to take the basement room, seeing as I had previously occupied the one at our previous house. To my surprise, and later dismay, this decision to move into the basement bedroom was one that saved the very fabrics of my mental health.

The early memories made at this house were inherently good. My family appeared to be happy, healthy, and much more comfortable with the increased space that it provided. Sure, I was still grieving the loss of my childhood home. But eventually I had to come to terms that in order to grow personally, I needed to let go of the past and take control of where I found myself in the present. Had I the foresight of what was to come, perhaps I would have prepared myself for the future. This little bungalow would later represent a place of resentment, distress, and long-lasting damage.

Something was churning up from within me. A festering self-loathing and hatred of myself. It had only been a matter of moments since the conflict had occurred. As I turned the corner of the basement stairwell and made my way to my bedroom, I gripped the light frame of the wooden door and slammed it as hard as I could. As if that effort hadn't produced enough of a comment on how I had felt, I decided to repeat the action a couple more times for good measure. I paced back and forth in the middle of the room like a caged animal does at the edge of its enclosure. My blood was pumping so fast that I could feel each individual pulse travel from my temples to the tops of my feet. A light perspiration had accumulated atop my forehead.

"We are your parents! You are to respect us! End of story!" These words rang through my head as I masochistic-ly punished myself (emotionally) for what I had done. I had stepped out of line, so I thought. I should have simply agreed with their statements. They were

my parents after all. All of a sudden, without warning, a thought struck me, like a strike planted on the side of the face, as I concluded my previous commentary. "Don't be such an idiot! No one has the right to treat another person this way. Not even one's parents!" I began to delve into a destructive cyclone of mental gymnastics. I was cross referencing all of the history of what had just occurred and, in rudimentary fashion, was looking for some kind of miracle-point that had given favour to my reactions as being "normal". Normal? What a strange word. Who or what can possibly define what "normal" is? Is my life normal? Are my fears normal? Are my reactions to my parents normal?

The stomping of feet above me drowned out such notions temporarily. I could hear my mother sobbing through the ventilation shaft, pleading with my father to do something that would make an impression on me. While I am not quick to assume that she was requesting for me to receive a physical reprimand, I felt as though I was calculating every movement I could hear in the house, perhaps in order to anticipate a confrontation. In the end, my psychology was shrewdly working against me.

CHAPTER THREE

WHAT HAPPENS BEFORE ME

Amidst this time of childhood change, the entirety of my family's dynamic was undergoing some unique personal challenges. Shortly after moving into the Avalon house, both of my younger siblings began to display abnormal behaviours related to focus and self-discipline. This ranged from staying on task during coordinated efforts like cleaning the house to overtly disobeying requests to go to bed when the clock struck 10:00pm. While Liam did not display the most severe of these responses (most of which mainly impacted his academic performance during early primary school), my youngest brother Quinn had a particularly difficult time controlling his temper. Well before he had turned five years old and was eligible for enrolment in Kindergarten, Quinn had presented himself as an outgoing, strong-willed, and incredibly imaginative child. He presented himself as someone that was overflowing with energy. If one needed evidence, the constant rhythmic tapping of eating utensils upon walls was enough to garner convincing. One thing that he used to do often was take two ballpoint pens, mind you they had to be the exact same brand or model, and would pretend to fly them around the house. It was precarious. Absurdly blissful (and at times intrusive) noise would often pour from his mouth. These sounds would serve as an attempt to mimic fighter jet gunfire. This type of imaginative play would go on for hours. Due to my (then) lack of personal education on the matter, I now ponder in retrospect whether or not such a behaviour gave insight to his growing mental condition(s).

Alongside the trivial reflections of those games, the more negative symptoms of something trying were beginning to rise to the surface. Instead of using words, fists were substituted to solve a problem. Rather than utilize gentle discussion, vulgar threats were often shouted from obscene decibel volumes. To avoid these increasing crescendo-ing scenarios, I tended to stick to my place of isolation in the basement. It wouldn't completely remove the stimuli that could be felt in the house, but it was the best option I had at the time. I would wait until the screaming and pounding had ended to carefully make my way back up the stairwell and into the depths of No Man's Land. The evidence was written all over the walls, literally. Gouges could be seen up and down the corridor. Some could be identifiable as the result of an object being thrown against it. Others were too similar in size to be anything other than a human fist. It was clear that Quinn was suffering.

In what seemed like an overnight span, which certainly could not have been the case for my poor parents, both Liam and Quinn were prescribed various medications to help regulate their flurry of hyperactivity and attention-deficit disorders. With respect to my parents, they had no idea what Attention Deficit Hyperactivity Disorder (ADHD) and Attention Deficit Disorder (ADD) were. Both conditions tend to be co-morbid with one another, creating a molotov cocktail of complications for the areas of life on which they are hurled. I can't speak on behalf of the conversations that my parents had with the boys' psychologist, but I assume they were along the lines of "Without medication and proper adaptations at home, these negative behaviours will continue to persist". All that could possibly follow would be a "Hell yes! Let's get started" kind of response. It would not take much for a couple who were desperately seeking help to say "yes" to achieving some semblance of peace.

For Liam, the medication seemed to serve its intended purpose. It allowed him to focus more on school. It also allowed him to control his compulsive habits, which helped to foster more positive social interactions with others rather than hindering them. For Quinn however, the transition to taking medication was a living nightmare.

Quinn resisted this new routine with a dedication reflective of a highly trained United States navy seal. In particular, the foreign object having to be swallowed proved to be an enormous challenge, not just because of the physical discomfort, but also because of the mental toll it caused. Rather plainly, he would mention to my parents that the pills would make him feel "off" or strange. This strange feeling would later evolve into a more serious thought that plagued his mind: "What if the medication is changing who I am?" I remember feeling deeply sorry for my brother. I was sorry that there was not a simpler way for him to find a solution to his problems. Clearly, he was in dire need of some kind of revelation that would help him overcome this cognitive hurdle. He deserved to feel whole. Hence, he began to elude the fact that he had begun hiding pills in various areas around his bedroom. Such locations included the bottom drawer of his dresser underneath various piles of old clothes, up top his closet shelf pushed as far back to the wall as possible, and even in holes in the walls.

One day, things took a turn for the worse. It was time for Quinn's medications to be taken before school. He had risen out of bed far too late, had not eaten breakfast, and certainly did not have his backpack compiled and ready for departure. Liam and I had muddled our way through our own menial tasks, tuning out the growing frustration that was growing between my parents and their youngest child. To them, the answer was straightforward: take the pill and all of the problems will go away. With the clock "tick, tick, tick"-ing away, and Quinn continuing to apathetically prepare, their patience eventually wore thin. They both pleaded for him to swallow the capsule. Quinn, understandably refusing to do so for fear of gagging/throwing up and (more importantly) departing into a place of mental unfamiliarity, vehemently refused. Frustrations then turned into hurtful words. Hurtful words turned into physical retaliation. Physical retaliation turned into deeply-rooted emotional wounds. Standing at the entrance of his bedroom, I watched as my parents forcefully pinned my brother down and force feed him a pill with a cup full of water. The events looked like a water-boarding torture scene. Quinn gurgled and sloshed as my father held his jaw shut, hoping that in the heat of the moment that the pill would slide down his throat. The strangest part? I felt myself joining into the Orwellian 1984-like chants that had begun with my parents' actions. "Just take the damn pill!" "It's not that difficult!" "You're doing this to yourself!" I was on auto-pilot. The earlier feelings of sadness that I had felt were replaced by flashes of white hot, putrid anger. I was inadvertently taking on a significant portion of responsibility for what was happening in front of me. After what felt like an eternity, the seemingly possessed child lay on his back staring blankly at the ceiling. Tears were flowing down the sides of his face. He was exhausted from the whole ordeal. I asked myself whether something that had been so trivial had to turn into such a massive outburst. Instead of joining in with my parents, why didn't I decide to push them off of Quinn and denounce what they were doing? To this day, this moment has left a significant impact on my heart. I had failed him in that moment. I would never be able to comprehend or communicate these feelings to him until years later.

When the dust had settled, my parents made it appear as though their child-rearing practices were ethically acceptable. Justifications of all kinds were used to substantiate the aggression and confrontation that were necessary in order to "get the job done". In a way, I had been hypnotized by this rhetoric during my younger years. Rather than contemplate the possibilities of what responsible conflict-resolution actually looked like, I had been convinced that there was simply a black and white response to all things familial. This included understanding one's role in the family hierarchy and what punishment looked like for disobeying this accepted ideology. If I had experienced a bad day at school and didn't let it show until I got home, I would expect to get yelled at. If I accidentally broke a plate or dish by dropping it to the floor, I would be made to feel that I had broken a precious family heirloom worth millions of dollars. Not to mention the shame I had felt whenever I began to think of breaking free of this house-turned-prison. The relationship between parent and child(ren) was quickly becoming soiled the longer that time went on. There was an obvious double-standard of how we children were made to think about what a family was and how it was to function. Just how much of this standard was created as a result of my parents trying to retain composure of their household? Quite a bit, I believe.

As time went on, the disruptions to what should have been an ordinary childhood continued. Along with his previous diagnosis of ADHD, Quinn had been additionally diagnosed with having Oppositional Defiant Disorder (O.D.D.). With this pertinent new information, it served as a proverbial death sentence to any form of serenity that still existed within the household. For context, ODD is often described as a form of severe defiance towards those of whom possess some form of recognizable authority. This can include one's parents, teachers, and even law enforcement. Due to the nature and time in which ODD was identified in his life, Quinn struggled to distinguish between which of his behaviours were natural adolescent developments and which were those that had been influenced by the disease. After all, he was a young boy at the time attempting to find his social footing, as any child does. I have memories of Quinn grappling with this duality, and inquiring as to how his mind would attempt to put into words the things he was feeling. It's as if you could stare into his eyes and see the puzzle just seconds away from being solved, but realizing that the final pieces had either gone missing or had been destroyed altogether. How infuriating it would be to constantly sit on the edge of self-awareness! Looking back, it's awful to think of Mom and Dad's intervention practices as anything but fuel being added to Quinn's wildfire.

***

It was August once again, and I was beginning my annual rounds of questioning my sanity as the summer season came to a close. Mom and Dad would request that it be time to pack all of our belongings into our bags and to prepare the cabin for its seasonal hibernation. Upon learning of this task, I did what any kid who feared the loss of freedom would: I ran away. Taking a bike from the nearby garage, I would high-tail it to some of Mistusinne's most remote locations. The best options would consist of the vast network of paths that were connected to the Trans-Canada trail, or the many beaches that stretched well past one's standard vision capabilities. Certainly, a part of me had chosen to run away as an emotional reaction to my parents' wishes. I was a hormonal child, at the time. However, I was equally as terrified to return to the city for one good reason. I did not want to become subjected to whatever outlandish arguments and fights that would ensue. Mistusinne had offered me seclusion; an escape from the inevitable certainty that something awful was bound to happen. My inability to determine, and even promote, a camaraderie amongst my family members had begun to warp my understandings of what a "healthy" family looked like. Everywhere I looked, I saw different representations of normality that were being offered to others. I would see families playing at the local park, smiling and laughing with one another. Even my close friends who had come from broken families (caused by divorce) were still able to maintain relationships with their parents out of pure, centralized, unabashed love for the other. I began to distance myself from my parents. Not only did I disagree with how they were parenting, I resented them for preaching one kind of sermon and living in an alternate reality.

It was once we had returned home to Saskatoon that the problems started once again. They did so like clockwork. I remember the plank of wood for a door creaking and groaning against the weight of an angered body desperately trying to pry it open from the outside. An argument had erupted between my mother and I. Likely, it was caused by something simple such as leftovers going missing from the fridge, or perhaps I had thrown her way an aimless comment in an attempt to portray my emotional state of mind. Regardless, it had always been this way since moving into the Avalon house. If words failed to effectively make a voice be heard, violence and aggression were quickly enacted as the next best option. I had been on the outside of my parents' upset for quite some time, arguably because much of their attention was being put on Liam's and Quinn's diagnoses. It was only a matter of time before their attention turned towards me.

Truthfully, my mother and I have never had what could be considered a healthy relationship. What my mother lacked in height, she made up for in personality. Standing at approximately five-foot-six inches, Mom dressed in chic modern clothing and would dye her hair to stay with the times. A trend-follower at heart, she appeared to most people as someone who was socially aware of herself and what interests she had. She would be the type of person to tell you what she thought, regardless if it didn't cross her mind the repercussions of doing so. I would imagine that she had to learn how to navigate her role as a maternal figure in a house full of testosterone. To give credit where it's due, it could not have been easy to manage three young boys who were constantly getting in each other's business. Between taking each other's belongings, and determining whose turn it was on the backyard swing, perhaps it would have been easier to flip a coin and let chance make the decision. However, there are other components that add to the way in which our childhood was shaped.

As Dad continued to work within the industrial sector, he quickly gained rapport and respect amongst his coworkers and superiors for being a successful businessman. I would often overhear the conversations between my parents of the "million dollar jobs" that he had secured between the company and a partnering Potash mine. I was proud of my Dad in these moments. He appeared to be genuinely excited about these updates, and the mood in the house would lighten dramatically. Eventually, he accepted a job offer that promoted him to the rank of corporate business manager. Dad would leave the house earlier in the mornings and would return from work later in the evenings. Again, justifiable in the sense that with increased responsibility, more time would be expected of him. Despite these positive developments, Dad found himself travelling for business meetings and opportunities (whatever that looked like... I had heard rumours of Las Vegas casino parties and strange extracurricular excursions like airboat rafting in the Everglades) quite routinely. This left my mother to be the primary caretaker and disciplinary figure to us three children. Over time, I could sense that this was taking a toll on her. And rather than have the effects of a difficult day resolve themselves over a good night's rest, they seemed to carry over onto each other the very next day. In fact, her decisions to enforce rule and order were actualized in rather dramatic ways. Some days, if child rearing had proved increasingly difficult, she would eat dinner by herself on the couch and ignore the pleas of provisions coming from her children; a consequence for not listening to the exact specifications of desired behaviour. Other times, hurtful and insulting language was directed to us as some form of last-ditch effort to make us feel guilty for the conflict that had transpired. The methods and severity of these actions evolved to a point where confrontation was becoming much more physical and uncomfortable. I imagine that to anyone, it would prove hard to hold a civil discussion when another person is violating your personal space in such a demeaning way.

As I listened to my mother shriek from the opposite side of the barricade, I had not noticed the tears begin to run down my face. I had neglected to feel my heart wrench from an uncomfortable pulse rate. Living like this was nothing short of horrible. If it wasn't me on the end of such repercussion (for the most part, I had done what I could to avoid it as much as possible); it was my brother(s). I believe, to this day, that to some degree my brothers and I have built a sense of empathy for one another for having endured a similar rearing experience from our caretakers. From beyond the pinned door I could hear my mother state, "Just you wait until your father comes home". And for the next several hours, days even, the clock would "tick" with the same impotence as that of an inmate on death row, who is nervously waiting for their ticket to be punched. Upon his return it had felt as though

31

my father had emerged as a character playing the inquiring executioner, delicately working to extract a guilty confession from the accused. The whole process he used felt grimy. Being called to sit in the living room across from my parents (while my Mom played video/audio recordings of the events captured via her cell phone) felt like a cheap shot for Mom to gain favour over my father and his not being present at the time of the incident. In many cases, what was recorded was but a sliver of what had actually transpired. It was manipulative and tricky. Now, I know what you may be thinking. "Were you ever guilty to some degree?" And to that I would say "of course!". I had allowed my juvenile brain, and lack of pre-frontal cortex control, to enact my fight or flight responses. What this confession does not include however is the insurmountable condemnations I had of myself that plagued my every doing, especially following a conversation where my parents and I had been arguing. I was made to feel that I held sole responsibility.

It was moments like these that created a rift of mistrust and disrespect between child and parent. I began apologizing and taking accountability for my actions, yet reciprocation from the opposing party never occurred. Such events persuaded me to reflect on the thoughts of who I wanted to be in life. I wanted to be a person who, despite his natural human flaws, would work to refine himself into a quality man. I wanted to feel that regardless of the hostile environment I was raised in, that I could pour empathy, respect, and life into others. I even prayed and held faith that God could turn my battlefield of problems into a calm armistice. If it didn't happen in the moment, surely if were to happen soon. Looking back, I can only see the profound nature in how He works, and how the Lord was diligently preparing me for the very things that I needed to reach this personal goal.

My obsessive compulsive behaviours increased in prevalence when I was around the age of 7-years old. They began with comments questioning the quality of my clothing, such as the fear that sleeves or neck holes would be too tight and feel constricting to wear. Later on, the procedures of bathing or showering began to follow a strict format. Rinse with water first, lather with soap afterwards. Start with the left arm, then move to the right arm. Focus on the left leg, then to the right leg. Lastly, shampoo the hair. To conclude, spend approximately three minutes rinsing off excess suds with water. And that was just the cleaning routine. Drying off with a towel and brushing my teeth followed a similar, neurotic pattern.

As if morning procedures weren't enough, these structuring habits began to transcend into other extra-curricular activities. On one occasion, likely for a birthday or for Christmas, I had been gifted a LEGO set. As I tore open the cardboard box in sheer excitement,

I also slowed my pace enough as to place all of the intermixed pieces into categorical groups. Every station was specific to a type of piece in relation to its size, colouration, or purpose. I would skim the instruction manual multiple times before gaining the courage to start building the product, brick by brick. There was something about the order that the task promoted that felt stable. I had time to enjoy the building process and marvel at the intricacy behind the toy's engineering. Upon placing the last stud, I would take a sigh of contentedness and revel in my creation. Such a model was not to be played with. Instead, it was placed upon a desktop or shelving unit to be admired from afar. Figures were positioned in such a way that it was highly noticeable when something (or someone) had touched or moved the setup. Such acts of my brothers became more than a mere nuisance; it became a violation of my personal rights and property! Or so I thought…

While the rest of my family lived by the decree of "go with the flow", I lived by the personal doctrine of "expectations provide stability". How was it possible that someone could live their life with arms wide open to the inconsistencies of the world? From my perspective, it was preposterous to see anything other than outlining one's day through a series of bullet-point to-do lists to serve as an effective way to ensure success.

The dormancy of my anxiety symptoms lay in the shadow of these experiences. On the outside, I appeared quirky. Strange, even. On the inside, I was enacting safety structures to help mitigate the feelings of being overrun by my emotions.

CHAPTER FOUR

LOKI

In Norse mythology, the figure *Loki* serves as an important reminder of the incorporation of humour and laughter in one's life. However, despite the good intentions of the jester, it oftentimes saw Loki placed into the middle of some … precarious situations. Mind you, the ramifications of his experiences were excellent for teaching both young and old about the foundational moralities of the world. He still served in his trickster ways and was beloved by those who heard of his endeavours. Jonah, for the purposes of this recounting, is my Loki.

I had frequently searched for avenues of normalcy throughout my childhood in order to get but a taste of "good" that others were fortunate to have. I didn't need charity, but I needed someone to advocate for me. Luckily, I was fortunate enough to have struck friendship with another young boy in my Kindergarten year of schooling. Jonah's rambunctious, and at times chaotically devious, personality never failed to rouse within me a hearty laugh and childish smile. It seemed as though everything that a child was told were "right and wrong" were backward to him. Moreso, such distinctions were suggestions as opposed to rules outlined within a social code. Behind the locks of his curly, dirty-blonde hair were eyes that spoke of experiences that included his own forms of grief. He had been plagued by his own demons, some of which altered his family dynamic quite significantly. But it was his ability to chuckle through the madness that made him special and stand out from the crowd.

Together, we experienced the joys and stresses of our most formative early years. We navigated the experimental trials of learning basic reading, writing, and arithmetic at primary school, as well as how to socialize with others for the purposes of maintaining healthy relationships. This is not to say that we did not have our fair share of differences, however. In fact, we failed at that second curriculum quite often. I have vivid memories of us fighting on the playground, over trading cards of all things, and concluding the fight with an adornment of shared bruises on both body and fists. We fought like brothers would. Something may be said or done (that was not received well) and the effects of such a decision would consist of temporary periods of frustration. War wounds aside, we know that our vexations stemmed from the high standards we secretly held each other accountable to. It was a curious symbiotic relationship.

It was us against the world, Jonah and I. We continued to grow up indulging in the same extra-curricular interests as one another, mainly relating to television programs or video games. Either one of us who came to school equipped with the hottest new information regarding a pop-culture hit would be eager to spill the details to the other. We also endured the hardships of navigating school life together. Receiving poor grades was one thing, but forming coalitions against those we considered to be pretentious was a whole different ballgame. We weren't the most popular chaps in the class, and it must have felt like there were precautions to take in order to watch out for one another.

Occasionally, our after school hangout sessions would transition into overnight ones. There were a few occasions where our parents had allowed for sleepovers to occur, and I was keen on requesting it to take place somewhere other than my home (for obvious reasons). The best times were those that included boxes upon boxes of pizza and a carefully selected horror movie that was guaranteed to scare the shit out of us for weeks on end. But eventually, the shenanigans would settle into periods of deep conversation where our innermost perceptions of life were shared. We would discuss topics that ranged from religion, girls, and even hypotheticals that stirred our insights of reality and shed light into what truths were and were not. For the first time in my life, I had someone who served as a vital outlet to allow me to be an honest and authentic version of myself.

His family took me on as their own, treating me (and at times even titling me) as their child. Their genuine kindness and interest in me are qualities that I will never forget, nor take for granted. The one person in this family that stood out the most, other than Jonah of course, was his mother. From the day I had met her, her tranquil demeanour and welcoming presence provided me with much peace. I had been consumed by a confusing world, yet her presence was an antidote to the symptoms of fatigue. Intentional with her words, I remember her asking me questions about my own family, friendships, and interests. At times, answering some of these questions proved difficult, if not, impossible. It may have been easier to simply nod and accept her preconceived notions of my familial equilibrium. The conversation was never limited to "yes or no" responses. She always made it known that she wanted to invest into me as a person; she wanted to invest in who I was to become. With all of this in mind, it made complete sense as to how her son had been raised to hone such an empathetic heart. She had passed down a character trait whose value was worth far more than earthly possessions.

Over the years, I was periodically invited over to their house to partake in family dinners and celebrations. The sense of unity amongst those seated at the table was strong, and over time, I began to feel rejuvenated and energized by the overwhelming fondness that these people had for one another. Jokes were shared, alongside petty family quibbles, that entertained non-threatening jabs at one's ego. As a reactionary response, I was fully prepared to duck under the table and wait for knives to be thrown. It never happened. Instead, I sat happily in union with the group, basking in the genuine atmosphere that allowed my heart to feel safeguarded and respected. It felt as though it was something that my own family had desperately lacked.

Upon returning to my own home after a time of bliss and good nature, it was evident that there was a notable, noxious feeling looming in the air. From the exterior of the house, one could almost imagine a haze of discomfort reeking from the orifices of the windows and front door. I even experienced that peculiar feeling that one has when they return to a familiar place and recognize the smell that makes it distinct. It smelled heavy and relayed the musk of stained wood. As I removed my footwear and hung my jacket in the entrance closet, I would keep my ears carefully attuned to any commotion that was occurring around the corner from my obscured position. It was always important to gauge whether one had missed an altercation and was wandering into a potential minefield. No explosions? Good. Carefully take another step. It would be considered fortunate if upon my return that my parents ask of how the outing went. However, most times my arrival went unnoticed, their focus preferring to remain on whatever it was that they were doing before. A sense of apathy would emanate from the halls of the house, that is until I was able to enter the familiarity of my basement bedroom. It was down there that the air felt the faintest touch lighter. It provided me a laboured breath of relief.

I look back on these moments with remorseful sentiment. The one place that a child should feel secure in is in their own home, and I was not feeling so. On top of this, the abusive nature of this childhood encouraged my brain to convince itself that I was overreacting; that I was manipulating myself into thinking that I was suffering. Often, these cyclical thoughts would be interrupted by pieces of the ceiling tile crumbling and falling onto my face. A confrontational match was occurring in the kitchen located directly above. Slurs and curses could be heard vibrating off of the house's foundation, filling every vacant space within it a negative energy. As I got older, I learned to place my iPod earbuds in, and play ambient music that could take me away from it all. Something needed to give. But even with music blaring into my eardrums, the shudders of the house would continue to bounce off of my skin, reminding me that escape was never truly an option.

As for Jonah, his and my story continued to evolve over time. Following graduation from high school, we both enrolled at the local university (University of Saskatchewan); myself interested in pursuing a degree in education, and he, a degree in psychology. We were both desperately single, and our lifelong companionship and free time had encouraged us to find space within our changing schedules to invest in one another. From time to time, we would meet at the campus racquetball courts and challenge each other to a friendly match. We would meet at the campus food court and talk (about nothing important in particular) for hours at a time. There were even rare occasions where we were able to identify common credits that we both needed to complete our respective programs.

As such, we would eagerly time our enlistments to ensure that we could piggy-back a course with one another. Nevertheless, as I eventually transitioned into my professional college at the start of third year, my studies saw me travel inter-provincially for an internship. This distance put between us made it difficult to be present in our friendship like I had before. Moreover, Jonah began to struggle with his own academic drive. His Loki-like behaviour would oftentimes encourage him to skip class and put precedence on other things with tantalizingly higher individual value. I made the critical mistake of allowing my unmindfulness to evaluate his choices in a negative limelight. It was highly unfair and largely influenced by a critique that had been mimicked in my home throughout most of my formative years.

I, on the other hand, continued to enjoy the difficult nature of post-secondary schooling. This is not to say that it was never difficult. It was. I acutely remember sitting behind a desk in one of the crammed university gymnasiums writing a geology final examination. I had studied for hours on end in preparation for it, only to be baffled at the document asking me what paleo-age an extinct form of parasite had originated from. None of the content that was covered in the course had even referenced this type of information. I ended up receiving a 51% on that very test. Yikes. Despite that, having an observable goal, like getting a degree, had made sense to me. It allowed for another channel to vent my personal problems of home, and better yet, gave me a way to get out of that miserable house.

Remarkably, Jonah has remained a consistent component of my life. While I can admit to the feelings of guilt for not staying in touch as much as I used to, our encounters have always been sparked by tacit memories and fastened experiences. Jonah still lives in Saskatoon and has become quite the impressive entrepreneurial artist, acquiring a niche following of illustrator admirers who commission him for unique pieces. In the end, my greatest hope is that he knows how much I value our friendship. He may never know it, but Jonah may well be the person who saved me from becoming a terrible person, as a result of unkempt personal standards. He may be unconventional, and even an eccentric at times (I'm sure he would agree), but he is the perfect amount of unconventional to keep you reminded of one greatly important lesson to learn in life: life is short. Don't spend it tied down to the expectations that you think you are bound to. Loosen up and learn to laugh a little.

The long hallway teemed with students of all kinds. Athletes, musicians, bookworms, gamers, actors, and the lot all mingling and hovering about. There was a potent hum of energy bouncing from within the confines of this locker-gauntlet. From a bird's eye view, the chaos surely would have resembled a colony of ants crawling overtop of one another, mindlessly moving to and fro. I clutched my school binder close to my chest and braced for the impending impact of others' unwary shoulders and backpacks. My chest tightened and breathing quickened. A noticeable drip of perspiration could be felt from my underarms.

"I just have to get to my seat," I thought. It was overstimulation. The noises of the typical school environment had amplified within my ears. The smells of different rooms would transport me back to specific memories, both good and bad. The worst was the math classroom. That scent was all too familiar. It was impossible to not succumb to the senses. At least once class had started, I could be somewhat distracted from the strange symptoms I was experiencing.

I had chalked up the sweatiness as a reaction to a deodorant stick I was using. Maybe the materials it was made of were irritants? The heart rate, however? That proved a little difficult to make an excuse for. Every one of my classmates appeared to be composed and focused. Some were rapidly scratching notes on their looseleaf papers. Why were they writing so quickly? Did the teacher mention an upcoming exam? "Goodness, I can feel a migraine coming on," I would tell myself.

.

CHAPTER FIVE
CAUGHT UP TO ME

According to the *Oxford English Language Dictionary*, the term abuse is defined as "[to] use (something) to bad effect or for a bad purpose; misuse". What stands out to me most in this description is specifically the word "misuse". Humans are prone to this form of behaviour. Some may blame mankind's natural curiosity to push the boundaries of the status quo. Others can note that certain individuals can identify the inherent power in manipulating their way into advantageous positions. With this in mind, it is not farfetched to consider that we live in a world that is simultaneously filled with both Renaissance thinkers and authoritarian dictators.

When I think back to my upbringing, in regard to my parents' child-rearing style, I don't automatically jump to conclusions about them being evil-natured. Surely, I would have to be wrapped-up in myself to ignore the many valid experiences that they themselves had gone through that had caused adversity. However, a common trend began to grow increasingly noticeable the older I became. My parents had created an intoxicating utopian image for our family unit; one that was not always authentic.

It is simple to understand the selfish desire to "put on one's best face" for public appearances. One wants to appear competent (confident even) about their role within the greater community and society in question. But at what point does doing so begin to warp one's internal ethics and morality?

Walking into the church foyer, following a vicious argument that had just occurred in the car, I could note my mother's plastered smile as she acquainted herself with the various eyes that intercepted the building's entryway. My father would be shortly behind her, prodding us forward with his forward-leaning posture and acute perception of our proximal distance away from him. Worship music could be heard blaring from the nearby auditorium speakers. We were late for service once again. It had become a regular pattern for our family over the years, and it was rare that our attendance was not marked by some form of underlying conflict. Nonetheless, my parents were clear in providing various non-verbal cues to us children about our required composure, so not to appear to other attendees as suspicious. Perhaps it is my personal understanding of the matter, but doesn't avoiding a confrontation allow for the bitterness to perpetuate itself? In retrospect, it was an absolute shame that us brothers weren't taught a more holistic form of conflict resolution.

I remember my agitations held towards my parents as they encouraged me to put aside my feelings for the duration of a church sermon and/or luncheon. It was yet another social appeasement, designed to allude the awareness of our fellow congregational members. From the pulpit, the pastor would deliver his messages of Christian virtues such as forgiveness, humility, and empathy. It was backed with scriptural reference about how some of God's most impactful people thrived in a life filled with religious persecution. Fuming with self-deprecation and contempt towards myself, I turned to view the faces of my parents who stared back blankly at the stage. I wondered if the Good News had made them feel any kind of remorse.

My relationship with the Lord had always been one of skepticism. For one, I had been raised in a household where Christianity was valued, but lacked consistent practice. Such a nuance stems from the fact that my father's side of the family are a batch of non-practicing Catholics. I categorize them as such not to prolong the centuries-long argument between Catholicism and Protestantism, but more so because it was highly difficult to discern what aspects of their lives were religious at all! Secondly, much of my knowledge about maintaining a personal relationship with Christ had come from the various conversations about the process in Sunday school. It begs to question how much of my childhood faith had been influenced by my parents and the faith that they had accepted.

And so, I tried to personalize my faith journey instead. I couldn't change the fact that I had been baptized as a newborn. Such an event had happened, and it ritualized the symbolic message of me being welcomed into the family of God. What I did decide to do however, despite everyone around me doing so, was wait to partake in the communion ceremony until I was emotionally ready for it. If baptism was viewed as an eternal induction into the "Christianity Hall of Fame", then the Lord's Supper was seen as the monthly playoffs. I faintly remember conversations being had between various similar-aged children at church and at school who had boasted about how young they were when they took the consumables (despite in the same breath mentioning how horrific their aftertastes were). And as I chuckled along with them in their self-satisfaction, I struggled to find my voice as to state how I really felt about their sacrilege. I chose to respect said persons who shared their insights with me, including my own brothers who began participating in the various Christian rights of passage. Although awkward to stay the only one sitting in the pew while the rest of the family went up to the stage, I felt like my decision to challenge my ownership of faith would serve as a foundational experience to reflect upon in the future. I can now look back in retrospect and say that this was definitely the case.

Life is not perfect. I have come to appreciate that everyone goes through their own experiences with the cards that they have been dealt. Nevertheless, the loss of perspective and compassion has been a destructive path that I have noted many of my family relatives to take. This path had been kept maintained through the lack of open conversation. It has also persisted due to the influence of social media and the various growing internet platforms. Instead of fostering a relationship through kindness, many have chosen to do so by turning a blind eye. As the days of my childhood turned to months, my emotional stability began to warp. In some circumstances, I found myself sympathizing with the whole ordeal; merely condoning what was happening because it was the best option to avoid putting a target on my back. In a way, I had become a spineless coward. I chose to selfishly look at my own interests, while others like my siblings, underwent the same kinds of exposure to trauma that I had (was). There were many moments of laying on my back in that cold, reclusive bedroom, noting the pieces of ceiling tile dust fluttering down to the mattress like falling snow. To me, having a speck of dust in the eye seemed far less painful than the types of emotional hurts that I was feeling.

Statistics (researched by many academic and widely respected institutions such as the *Center for Disease Control* [C.D.C]) state that stress and anxiety are the leading causes of both physical and mental health deteriorations in younger age demographics. Such factors are the reason why many people nowadays are diagnosed with an assortment of medical conditions like high blood pressure and cardiovascular disease. It truly is a pandemic of the non-contagious variety. It also persists to be a widespread issue that is misunderstood by those who have never had to deal with the effects of such conditions. For the longest time I had told myself that I was not a part of these statistics. I was going to fight against all of what had been placed before me. I would not be a casualty.

I eventually lost that fight.

The old man solemnly stared at us as he remained slumped from within the confines of his La-Z-Boy recliner chair. The room was constricting and deafeningly quiet. A static hum existed, despite the lack of audible noise from within the living quarters. I looked over at Dad, hoping that he knew of some way to make the situation less uncomfortable. However, most questions asked of the old man were responded to with a sloth-like paced head nod. It was difficult to get any form of verbal communication out of him.

My father had driven my family down to Regina (two hours south of Saskatoon) one summer when I was approximately thirteen-years-old. He had been given word from my Grandma Santha that his Grandfather Donald was deteriorating at a rapid rate. He was becoming increasingly frail. Thus, when my Great Grandfather turned the corner of ninety-years-old, it served as a solid opportunity for my family to celebrate this milestone alongside the rest of my Dad's extended family. Additionally, it allowed for an opportunity to let us kids meet this strange character that we had never heard of before.

Regardless of our lack of knowing him personally, my father assured us that Donald was a good man. Aged, but good.

After entertaining a few one-sided conversations, Dad asked his Grandfather a question in the most delicate of tones.

"Grandpa, do you think we can go see the basement?" The old man's eyes shifted dramatically upwards to meet my father's. It was the fastest bodily reaction that I had noticed of him so far during this visit. After contemplating the question for what seemed like a dramatic minute, Donald hoisted himself up and out of the recliner and slowly inched his way through the kitchen, towards the basement stairwell. Dad motioned for us kids to quickly follow suit, and we watched as the old man nervously made his way down the stairs, one feeble step at a time, one hand lynched around a handrail. Whiskey and rum bottle caps lined the slanted roof as it made its descent into the lower part of the dwelling. I would later be told that Great Grandpa Don and his drinking buddies would take each bottle cap and glue it to the ceiling as a reminder of the good times that were had. There must have been hundreds of them.

Once Donald reached the bottom of the shaft, he reached to flick on a nearby light switch, which quickly illuminated the otherwise unnerving cavern of darkness. The light had given way to a series of doorways; one that led to a laundry room, one to a small storage closet, and the other to a large den that resembled the likes of an early 90's billiards room. The neon liquor signs, standup barstool, and snooker table would sell the attitude of this space if the faint musty smell did not. Donald peered towards the den, and for a short moment, paused in what seemed to be a stint in his consciousness before turning to my father. He slowly pat Dad on the stomach and returned back up the stairs. Not a word was spoken. The retreat had felt strange, but I shrugged the moment off as my attention was caught by something else that had been gleaming from the corner of my eye. Encased within a glass cabinet were a series of meticulously placed war medallions, caps, and documents. Each piece was labelled with the name of my Great Grandfather and reinforced in its authenticity with a picture of a young man dressed in his army regalia. Donald was a veteran of the Second World War.

As we continued to explore the growing world of the old man's "man cave", the tone of our excursion would dramatically shift with the motioning of us kids to meet by one of the walls located closest to the den's entryway.

"Great Grandpa said that it was okay for me to show you this," Dad said as he fumbled with the cordage that secured a roll of textile to a fastener, not one foot below the surface of the roof. As the rope was unwound, he slowly allowed the canvas to roll towards the floor, revealing the stark red, white, and black colours of a swastika-laden Nazi flag. My brain stopped functioning. My eyes began to scan the relic, noting the light wear and tear that existed along the edges of the fabric material. It was also impossible to not recognize the characterizing reddish-brown stains of blood that littered the surface of the Aryan banner.

"He was a fuel tank operator for the Allies in World War II," my father started. "One day as he was making his way out into the field, his vehicle was targeted by an Axis bomber strafing run. Grandpa managed to dive out of the driver's side door just before the gunfire and munitions had reached the tank. He had nowhere to go. With pistol in hand, he ran towards the nearest German tank, pulled open the latch on its top, and took out every man that was inside. He took this flag from that machine, along with a Luger and rifle. The rest is difficult to get out of him".

The story imprinted itself on my mind with such ferocity that it continued to play even after the flag had already begun to be rolled back up into its hibernation pose. I pictured my Great Grandfather, albeit in younger (more athletic) form, doing the seemingly impossible.

Not only had he volunteered to serve in the war effort, but he had followed through on his promise and committed acts that appeared to the common-man as impossible to do. He was a hero.

Great Grandpa Don didn't talk much once we came back up from downstairs. Something in his face had changed. His eyes appeared even more sunken in than before, and his conversations could not be pieced together as coherently. He was shellshocked, even decades after the incidents in which his traumas had originated. How strong he had to be in order to live with these mental demons plaguing his sentience. I had never met the man before, yet I felt connected to him through the knowledge of the power of one's psyche.

SEAS OF YELLOW

CHAPTER SIX

LILAPSOPHOBIA

In Grade 5, I experienced my first major panic attack. Now, I had known by this point in my life that I had struggled with some form of irregularity concerned with my anxiety. But I was unsure of just how extreme it could become. As such, the physiological conditions I was suffering from (which includes profuse sweating, zoning in and out of consciousness, and vexation of paranoias) had to be carefully monitored. With no one at home to take my matters seriously, it was up to me to keep everything under control.

These attacks typically began with a standard experience; my hands would become clammy and I would notice my attention start to drift away from anyone and anything within the near vicinity. Next, my unconscious would apply the very worst possible outcomes to the circumstances that I was hyper focused on. If it had something to do with crowds, I imagined that I would be pushed to the ground and trampled to death by the feet of apathetic passersby. If I was swimming, I pictured diving to the bottom of a pool to retrieve an object and be unable to break the surface of the water for air. If it was a hospital or doctor's office-related activity, I envisioned receiving a diagnosis of a terminal form of cancer. I would transport myself to the scene of a hospital room, where I was positioned into a "death pose" on the patient bed, feeling every ounce of life draining from within my body. Maybe these thoughts weren't as much dramatic as they were creative.

One fateful afternoon, I had been sitting in my classroom attempting to write a math exam that focused on the solving of improper fractions. For not liking math, it is quite curious to note that certain terms can evoke a long-lasting primal fear in one's memory. Like that of "SOHCAHTOA". Even now I shudder at the brief thought of it. Any-who, math had never been my strong suit, but I had grown to profoundly respect my teacher who taught it, Mrs. LaPlante. Irrespective of my dreadful ability to work with numbers, I wanted to impress her that fateful day with how much I had studied and prepared for the test. She was unlike other teachers who merely wanted to have their students sit down for an hour and stay quiet. She taught the curriculum with knowledge and grace. In previous years, I could note how my teachers would grow increasingly fatigued from the assistance I required to comprehend basic arithmetic. However, Mrs. LaPlante was able to single-handedly crush most of my negative experiences by meeting me on my level. She empathized with my feelings.

As the graphite pencil scratched away at the paper before me, I could begin to note a rattling sound that started to echo from within the far corner window of the room. From beyond the glass-pane, a large, black, imposing storm cloud was seen quickly approaching the school property. Due to the brewing weather system, doubled with the test anxiety that I was already experiencing at hand, I began to feel my breathing rate increase and my palms secrete sweat. My face then turned flush, my hearing disappeared, and all of the consciousness that I had procured was obliterated. I tried to mask this concern by thrusting my arm into the air, a gesture that implied I needed help (only this time it was for reasons other than math). Mrs. LaPlante became aware of my request and gently came to my desk side to provide assistance. To be completely honest, everything that occurred after this moment is but a blur to me. I remember the school bell ringing, my peers making their way outside for lunchtime recess, and me hyperventilating in the classroom with my teacher at my side. As I convulsed in my seat, gasping for air, tears running down the sides of my face, I remember Mrs. LaPlante talking to me in the lightest voice imaginable. She began rubbing my back between the peaks of my shoulder blades and mentioning that she was "with me". When I came to, I was horrendously embarrassed. Was a math test and a spring storm really bad enough for me to react in such a way? I must have looked so incompetent and immature. At this point in my life, I was already incredibly self-deprecating. Additionally, self-efficacy had proved already difficult to achieve in middle school as it was.

That day marked my awareness of dealing with a true phobia. I was afraid of tornadoes. Funny, right? I even chuckle out loud anytime that I genuinely consider this reality. And although I had just undergone an outburst in class, I was not aware enough to know that this fear had been actualized on a day that preceded it.

That previous summer, my parents had taken us out to the cabin to live there for the two months as per tradition. As a result of being away from the city for such extended periods of time, it meant that my brothers and I were quickly falling behind on various extracurricular milestones. The most pertinent one? Acquiring our swimming level competencies and certifications. My parents had good reason to be concerned with this matter, as swimming in an open body of lake water proved to have more potential dangers than that of a supervised indoor pool. Luckily for us, swimming lessons were being offered right within the village of Mistusinne! A local family had decided to attain employment through the Red Cross foundation, and were given permission to host lessons in Lake Diefenbaker itself. From an evaluative perspective, this was the best-case scenario for a young boy such as myself. I had already become well acquainted with the cold and unpredictable waters of the lake due to years of previous beach excursions. By default, proving my swimming abilities to the instructor should prove relatively simple.

One morning, I woke up to the sound of the aspen trees violently blowing from outside of my bedroom window. As I nervously lifted the blinds away from the wall, I could note the opaque, evil clouds swirling from overtop my sleeping quarters. It was swimming lesson day, and Mom was certain that we would attend, stormy weather or not. Needless to say, I began to grow increasingly uncomfortable with the thought of doing so in such conditions.

"Mom, I think I am going to skip swimming lessons today. The weather outside doesn't look too good, and I'm starting to get an upset stomach," I debated.

"It looks fine outside. They won't make you swim in bad weather," Mom replied. This posed as an immediate problem to me. It appeared as direct dismissal. As I reluctantly made my way to the car, sit with skull pressed hard into the headrest, and watch out the window as we drove towards the beach, my mind became less focused on learning new floatation techniques and more on what was up above the water. From across the lake, lightning began to touch down on the vacated farmer's fields.

"Levi, hurry up! It's time to get in the water!" Mom yelled. Standing at the shore, I looked back and forth, from water to the sky, hoping that my hesitation would allow my case to gain some merit. I was stalling for time, albeit I was legitimately afraid. The wind began to pick up and the lightning and subsequent thunder strikes grew closer with every growing second.

"I can't do it!" I shouted, hoping my voice could be heard above the howling of the wind. I crossed my arms and planted my feet firmly in the sand. It wasn't going to happen. What happened next would burn deeply into my insecurities for the years to come. Mom began to laugh at me. I started to sob, the tears from my eyes mixing with the rain that began to drop onto the beach. It was a cruel moment of unfiltered emotional abuse.

I never did go in the water that day. Instead, I decided to run all of the way back to the locked cabin barefoot, lamenting about what had happened down at the lakefront just moments prior. Upon their return from lessons, which did intersect with a torrential downpour, I was treated with shame and guilt for wasting time and money. To this very day, storms and tornadoes continue to have this strange impact on my behavioural reasoning. Some days, I am hypercritical of myself and this self-imposed irrational fear. Other days, I am reminded of the wet pavement underneath my feet, and the mop of wet hair atop my head as I trekked back home with a beaten down ego.

After Mrs. LaPlante was able to calm me down to a reasonable level, she gave me a hug and walked down the hall with me to the school's vending machine. Out of her own wallet, she bought a ginger ale and offered it to me as a way to reinforce her genuine support. As if that wasn't enough, she chose to spend her lunch hour eating with me in the classroom to talk about non-relevant things to lift my spirits. She was a saint. I am grateful to reflect upon these moments and know that people like her were in my life. In reality, she likely had no context as to why such a reaction of mine had been evoked by a mere storm. Instead, she selflessly took the situation at face value and decided to play the role of a good person. If only there were carbon-copies of this woman, and that they were able to help us through all of our problems. I understand that it is not necessarily realistic to wish for instant tranquility in the "real world", but was she ever good at attempting to replicate that feeling to others as much as possible.

My adolescent years had marked the start of a rocky realization: I was not properly equipped to deal with change and stress. At home, the message was quite clear.

"Everyone deals with stress. Figure it out and get over it," as my Dad would put it. My anxiety continued to pop up from time to time throughout my middle school and high school years, but perhaps I was able (or learned) to mask it well enough to not make it appear as noticeable as before. Maybe instead of letting it out at school, I simply took it home and let it spew there instead.

---≈---

"Hellooo! How are you!? Come on in!" the jovial voice rang out. It was a warm, fateful day in September, and my brothers and I were prodded by our parents through the front door of an Ultracuts barbershop. All three of us siblings were donning similar overgrown hairstyles that badly needed to be tamed. So, for sake of ease and cost, my folks had identified this small hole-in-the-wall shop that could offer the needed services quickly and affordably. The bustling hairdressing studio smelled of a combination of rich hair product and middle-aged women's perfume. Littered across the floor were shavings from what must have been dozens of previous patrons. Lastly, lined within their seats, like cattle at a feed trough, were older women chatting away with their stylists. For a kid, it was a weird environment. If not weird, it was definitely overstimulating. Nonetheless, we required our obscured vision to be cured before returning to school in the coming days.

Having become acquainted with the business' features, my family's attention was redirected by the charming personality of a smiling

Chinese woman quickly approaching the front booking desk.

"Well look at these handsome young men you have here!" she exclaimed. She had raised her arms wide in the air, almost as if gesturing that she was welcoming a hug. Her cheeks shone with the colour of light red roses, and her dimples made it difficult not to smile back at her humbling compliments. She introduced herself as "Julie". One by one, my brothers and I were called to her back chair to climb atop a leather booster seat. With a couple pumps of the hydraulic foot pedal, Julie was able to raise our heads to her shoulder height. And without much warning, she would swiftly enter into thorough conversation, covering the various bases of discussion that ranged from academics to personal hobbies to school crushes. All the while she would rigorously toss our mangled hair to and fro until it positioned itself into a place where it could be lobbed off with a pair of scissors. I'm quite certain I had (at times) checked to make sure that she hadn't taken any of my ears off during the commotion! I had never talked with a hairdresser so much before, and it worried me that such exchange could potentially result in me receiving a bowl cut hair style. To my surprise, it was completely the opposite. Julie was a master at multi-tasking.

Haircut appointments continued on as such for several years. What started out as menial conversations soon turned into sessions where Julie was providing advice for our own circumstances in life, most of which were based on her own personal experiences. It became quite clear that she was looking to invest in her clientele. She wanted to know the good, the bad, and the ugly. It is what truly set her apart from the rest.

Julie has, and continues to be a constant in my life. In the days before I took my driver's exam, she was there to tell me to make complete stops at streetlights and stop-signs. In the days before I walked my university convocation stage, she was there to empower me in the work it took to get to that place of accomplishment. In the days *before my wedding, she was there to proclaim that love is the best feeling one can experience in a lifetime. Of course, the haircuts were a bonus.*

When life began to increase in difficulty, Julie had remained a personal life-coach. A hard-working woman, it was always in her nature to be on-call for an appointment scheduling opportunity. Although she would never admit it, I was always quite aware that she would sneak me in during a fictional time slot that didn't even exist (well after her shift had already ended). On top of that, I would note the lack of a personal monetary tip on my payment receipts. So, in subsequent sessions, I would ask for the debit machine in advance so that I could add a bonus for her on top of the standard bill. I was no match for her cunning wit. As we finished up our usual conversations, she would thumb the machine's buttons using rote memory (away from my eyes and general awareness) to avoid the tipping option. Sneaky! The most important rule to knowing Julie is to never question her methods.

***

"Hello, Levi! Come on in!" Julie was finishing up with another client, and I was ushering the little feet of a two-year-old to the nearest vacant chair in the waiting area of the shop.

"How are my boys doing?" she inquired. "Looking as handsome as ever!" she would follow-up. As the years passed, my hair had come and gone as the result of genetics. Yet the loss of it did not cease the relationship I had maintained with the friendly hairdresser. As my son began to climb up the barber's stool, I could not help but see a remarkable reflection of myself in the way that he conversed with Julie. There was talk of dinosaurs and his favourite things to do with Mama and Papa. And as they continued to interact with one another, I would glance down at my phone and the previous text message that

had confirmed our appointment. My initial text read:

"Hi, Mom! Do you have any openings available within the next coming weeks?" What followed was the reply:

"Happy Tuesday, Son! I have a slot ready for this Thursday".

CHAPTER SEVEN

DOG DAYS OF SUMMER

Picture the timeless scenes of sailboats on the open water, rhythmically rocking from the waves that crash against their starboards. Next, imagine the ripples of horizon-line heat mirages, sizzling atop their asphalt roadways and causing onlookers to wonder of the science behind the phenomenon. Finally, visualize two kids having one adventurous-as-hell summer work experience, with thrills a plenty!

"I'm going to climb the tree and touch one!" Brent exclaimed as he rolled out of the moving Ford six-wheel Gator.

"If boss man hears of this, we are going to be in SO much trouble!" I replied nervously. I sat in the cockpit of the vehicle, nervously tapping my fingers on the steering wheel, as I watched my coworker bushwhack his way through crowds of thorn shrubs and spiders' webs. Surely, this was to be another moment for the childhood memory books.

In the summer of 2010, I acquired a job as a seasonal maintenance worker at the Resort Village of Mistusinne. I was relatively new to the work world, and like many other youths, had been looking to make some money during the summer break and acquire some professional work experience. It just so happened that such an opportunity became available at this already-beloved location of mine. My father was the one who originally heard of the job posting, and referenced the online listing to me. It was a dream come true.

The two summer student positions were eventually filled by myself and another young man by the name of Brent. Brent came from a large, lively Catholic family, himself being lodged somewhere in the middle of them all. He had a bright personality, was goofy, and was also an endearing storyteller. In fact, his characteristics appeared much like what I had come to know of my childhood friend Jonah as having. As a result, it did not take long for the both of us to become friends. Much of our earliest conversations occurred during the monotonous duties of our assigned work tasks.

The work itself was nothing to gawk at, however. It consisted of cleaning isolated garbage bins and hauling them to the larger community waste bins, line trimming around every fencepost and roadway, mowing the golf course fairways, etcetera. But despite these humbling responsibilities, there were many other moments along the way that proved to be more difficult than anticipated. Working an outdoors job meant that one was constantly exposed to the glaring sun above, which lasted from a seasonally-extended sunrise to sunset. Ask any local, and they could tell you that there isn't a kind of heat quite the same as a dry Saskatchewan heat.

The difference this feature had on me could be easily noted in my "before and after" photos of the summer months. I was like a piece of white bread that had been left in the toaster for too long.

In between the cleaning of public washrooms and the pruning of overgrown saplings, Brent and I were trained on how to operate the machinery and equipment of the maintenance department. All it took was a completion of a *WHMIS* assessment, and probationary observation shift, and we were set to begin our two-month mission. At times, I couldn't help but smile as I twisted and turned atop the zero-turn mower. I realized that I was being paid to have so much fun. Other times, I questioned my decision to submit a resume for the job, as I was slowly being cooked alive in the sweltering heat of the ditches that housed multiple flower beds. Regardless of the coincidentals, this job proved to be a positive benefit to my mental health. I was able to wake up early each morning, before anyone else was even remotely close to doing so, and bike to the shop through the brisk fog. The bike route offered a complete aversion to any form of unwanted conversation or drama. I could work all day and return home with a couple of new cuts and bruises, which served as excellent conversation pieces about the victories that were had. On some occasions, I would even have enough time in the evening to bike straight down to the beach and plunge into the water to rinse off all of the dust and sweat that I had accumulated throughout the day. Paradise is what it was.

Now, Brent and I had very different interpretations of what strong work ethic looked like. Don't get me wrong, there were a handful of times where he worked incredibly hard to do something that was physically demanding (and I sat on the sidelines, watching like a proud father watches his son). However, he also knew how to take it easy and make a boring moment anything but. I had noticed this type of behaviour from the day I met him. In front of other adults, he was attentive; social even! Alone, with no direct supervision, his free-spirited nature was free to reign. In all honesty, I was quite worried about being lumped together with him due to proximity and association, should my efforts be questioned. So, I would spend hours of those first few weeks working by myself, doing the jobs that the other employees loathed. The worst of them all had to have been weeding the plant beds. Thousands of black flies and no-see-ums would swarm, craving the opportunity to suck the blood from your sweat-stained skin. But by around mid-summer, other tasks saw Brent and I work together for the sake of ease. It also allowed for the fostering of camaraderie.

One blisteringly warm day, Brent and I, accompanied by another local and friend of the maintenance department, took a jet ski out onto the lake and secured a floating swimming platform to an anchor submerged at the bottom of the water. The water was rather inviting, and the chance to break the monotony was welcomed. On a different day, we took the rusted-out, beat-down Ford work truck and spread mulch around tree beds all across the entirety of the village. We would chat with one another about family life, school, and even philosophy. Although, I cannot speak confidently about the profoundness of said conversations. Last but not least, there was one special day where Brent had decided that it was time to have some extra fun.

The two of us had been driving a pile of dead brush to a compost pile located at the west end of the village. Upon our return trip back to the shop, Brent had noticed an eagle's nest perched in the heights of some nearby poplars. He thrust up a mighty parley concerning how "cool" it would be to become a falconer and maintain a bond with an animal whose original intents were to remain wild. Whether he was exaggerating or not, I was unsure. Yet, he certainly made a case for the hypothetical by the sheer excitement of the idea alone. It was then that Brent had suddenly skipped off of the side of the John Deer, stumbling his way to balance, and sprinting into the trees towards the nest. Within a moment, he had already begun to assume the position of a bear cub trying to paw its way up to the top of a tree canopy.

"If you fall and hurt yourself, I am not assuming any responsibility. I hope you know that!" I yelled after him.

"Don't worry man, I'll grab a chick for you too!" he replied, predominantly focused on the task at hand and chuckling at the nuance the comment had to me still being a single guy. When he finally reached the top of the tree, he peered into the nest and spectated the life that was being housed within it. As I sat in the vehicle from a distance, I couldn't help but be intrigued towards Brent's approach to life. Here he was, at work, goofing off and doing things that he likely shouldn't be. He didn't seem concerned, however. In fact, upon telling the act of heroism and bravery to our boss in-person, he received a volley of laughter and applause. I laughed alongside the recounting, shocked that our boss had not felt mortified of learning about the stunt.

That same week, both our boss and another senior employee were scheduled to take a trip out of the village for the day. They had needed to acquire various parts to repair one of the mowers, and as such, had to travel to the nearest retailer. Both men mentioned to us that we were the only staff in the village that day, and were trusted to take good care of the facilities in their absence. We agreed, of course, and wished them well as they drove out and away from the yard. To me, it seemed to be just another day on the job. To Brent, it was an opportunity to be mischievous.

We spent the morning performing our regular tasks of cutting the greens, cleaning up garbage, and watering the shrubs. In spite of the normal state of affairs, as lunch time rolled around, Brent approached me with an enticing idea. He had noticed over the past several weeks that the one senior employee had been living out of an RV on the maintenance shop site. Later that summer, that same crew mate would confirm this living situation as being a temporary solution to his permanent residence being located far from Mistusinne. Attached to the back of his RV was a small propane grill, practically begging for someone to use it. After listening to Brent's initial plea of how hard we had both worked that morning, and how there were some leftover Canada Day beef patties inside the work freezer, he conjured up the idea to borrow his dad's propane tank and use it for a cookout. At some point mid-conversation, I decided to go along with it. We both hopped onto the Gator and cruised our way to his cabin, and proceeded to steal the tank off of his parents' back porch and hook it up to the grill back at the RV. I remained incessantly reluctant about the plan, despite going along with it. I kept a close eye on our perimeter, in the odd chance that our fellow staff made an unprompted return. The entire time, Brent housed a massive grin across his face. I was once again floored at how he could feel so carefree about it all.

Flashes of my anxiety had ignited sporadically during these times. For one, the summer storms had not stopped just because I had acquired a job that was outdoors. My body was still experiencing the mental and physical effects of stress, such as the migraines, shortness of breath, and even conscious lapses in judgement/awareness. Unsure of what was happening at the time, I chalked it up to being food poisoning or perhaps a stomach bug that was passing through family members in the cottage. On days where I had a lot of time for my mind to sit and wander, which happened often due to the nature of the job, these responses would flare up with consistent intensity. I was rapidly losing the ability to maintain control of these emotional surges. To make matters worse, there were still issues happening at home that I was not able to elude. Distress and irregularity had become a prevalent factor of my life.

At the end of August that summer, I said my goodbyes to Brent and the rest of the crew of the maintenance department. And as I hung my set of work keys on its rack and closed the door to the shop, I couldn't help but look back and reminisce on all that had happened. I had worked hard, made some solid money for the upcoming school year, and even made a new friend. Life was good. But much like it had before, summer was ending. It was time to return to the city for another round of high school.

I never did see Brent after that last day together. I don't know if he moved somewhere else, if he got married, or if he became a trained falconer. What I do know is that he taught me a valuable lesson that I won't soon forget. That to lose your sense of happiness and carefree attitude, amidst the confines of life, is to give up the gift of living in the moment. Since I was a child, I had become attuned to fitting into the various moulds of life. Much of my informal education had been focused on not messing up and paying the price of ignorance. Much of how I operated was due to my attempts to avoid conflicts with my parents, as well as the supposed others whom I was told would critique me in a similar manner. I had been provided a life that was built on a foundation of sand. It shifted and eroded over time.

I don't think I ever would have taken Brent's advice to climb a fifteen-foot tall tree, nor to steal another man's propane cylinder. But the general approach to life that he was living by, one of confidence and authenticity, was one that I could see myself getting behind.

---≈---

"GAH!" I suddenly gargled awake, choking on the saliva that had accumulated in my throat during the first few hours of sleep. I sat myself upright, albeit hunched over into a weak ninety-degree angle. My eyes scanned the room rapidly. My attention would quickly fixate onto the irregular noises that were exuding my mouth; those caused by a series of hurried, laboured breaths. Not again...

"Is this real? Am I really awake?" I wondered. I would proceed to hold my outstretched hand in front of my face, flipping it from front to back, as if to determine that it was in-fact my true conscious self. The red glare of the digital clock on my desk displayed the digits "03:27AM". Disappointed at the machine, I crashed backwards onto the bed and let out a sigh of frustration. Another nightmare had taken over the few precious moments available in the day to acquire rest.

How I longed for the stereotypical nightmare where one found themselves in a public place, dressed in nothing but a revealing pair of underwear. Better yet, I would have even opted for a dream where

I was mugged in an alleyway by a pack of dangerous thugs. To my misfortune, my dreams were almost always related to a form of family quarrel.

The details of these dreams were remarkably similar. And although the environments would differ between them, the dialogue amongst the characters involved was always the same. There was no transition between cordial communication and blatant screaming. It was always 0-100. The strangest part is that there remained a faint awareness of meta-cognition within the dream sequence itself. The expectations of the story would unfold with foreseeable climaxes and conclusions.

Real life was bleeding into the fictional. This sleep paralysis demon was one of different cognitive properties. I prayed for peace. What would I have to do to turn my brain off for one night? Unable to fall back asleep, I would often turn myself over onto my side and listen to music through a pair of headphones just to level the "noise" that was ringing within my ears. The cracks and groans of the building's frame would remind me where I was. How eerie it was that the dark of night was the only intermission from the energy of the house's inhabitants.

The stomping of feet and slamming of cupboards would denote the waking hours of the day. The harsh sunlight was beginning to peek its way through the curtains of the basement windows. As my brain was reactivated by the provocations, I stared blankly at the patterned ceiling tile above. My eyes felt heavy and my limbs felt weaker than usual. A tear had traversed the realms of my dreams and now found itself rolling down the side of my cheek in the real world.

SEAS OF YELLOW

CHAPTER EiGHT

SAN PIETRO IN VINCOLI

In my freshman year I enrolled into an extracurricular program that involved international travel to the countries of Italy, France, and the United Kingdom. It was difficult to pass up on such an opportunity, not just because of the sheer euphoria that the itinerary illustrated, but also because of the surprising benefits that were included in the trip package. Such benefits comprised of pre-determined hotel bookings, tables at authentic traditional restaurants, expedited admittance tickets into cultural centres of importance, etcetera. The catch was that I would have to wait a couple of years until I was a senior (as that was the projected year of travel). I banked on the idea that school would keep my mind preoccupied enough to avoid the periodic feelings of restlessness as the days slowly counted down to departure. After all, the occasion was a no-brainer. So, I decided to commit by financially enrolling, using much of the money that I had saved up during my previous summer occupancies at Mistusinne to fund the venture.

At the start of April in 2014, myself, four student peers, a parent volunteer, and teacher chaperone met at the Saskatoon international airport in the early hours of the morning. Despite it being early springtime, the sky was still pitch black, and a noted vacancy of the premises could be identified by the lack of taxi cabs and noise. Baggy eyes and yawning aside, our tiny group of travellers were all excited to board the plane and make our efforts a reality. We checked our luggage in, had our carry-on bags examined, and secured our plane seats before the passenger jet took us down the tarmac until it launched headfirst into a waterfall of opposing gravitational force. This was it! All we had to do was transfer at Toronto Pearson airport and we would officially be flying overtop the Atlantic to our destination(s)!

There is something to be said about the enjoyment that can be had while getting to your end-goal target. In fact, countless memories were made between us students along the way. I remember lying prone on the dingy airport floor playing cards with one another; a perfect way to kill time in between the long stints of waiting. With limited group members involved in the trip, we were encouraged to talk to one another and form meaningful relationships, which never would have happened otherwise. One of my fellow travellers even lost their passport in the Frankfurt airport, opting to leave it at the helm of a cash register where, not moments before, he joyously bought a package of Belgian chocolate. The panic in his eyes when his full name was listed overtop the airport speakers was nothing short of hilarious. As was the mad scramble to search in his pockets for a document that was clearly missing. The recurring joke was brought up many a time when spirits needed to be lifted. As expected, we eventually made it to Europe after a long excursion that included an overnight flight. It was the kind where fellow passengers' snores would wake one up periodically. That didn't matter though. The trade off of insomnia for exciting anticipation was well worth it.

Shortly into our arrival, we were met by a friendly local tour guide, an Italian version of *Indiana Jones*, who instantaneously took us from historical feature, to cultural epicentre, to modern fascination. His personal knowledge of the sites we were exploring was inspiring. We walked the original cobblestone roads that lead straight to the arches that adorn the Coliseum. We paraded through the crowds of people that line the hallways of the Louvre museum. We ate fish and chips in a British pub that looked and sounded like the kind one would dream of experiencing. Perhaps it was due to the oversaturation of attention-grabbing stimuli that existed in these spaces, but Saskatoon felt like a small blip on my awareness of an ever-increasing, greater world.

In fact, I can confidently state that home rarely crossed my mind. Sure, the hotel sleeping arrangements left more to be desired as, in many cases, the rooms or hallways smelled like an open cigarette ash tray. Additionally, some of the French cuisine presented aromas that felt rather off-putting to my bland western palate. There were so many strange soups and meats. Exquisite, yet foreign. On second thought, maybe I did miss the simplicity of a grilled-cheese sandwich… Nonetheless, the enchanting nature that comprises the views of the Tiber River, Eiffel Tower, and Big Ben proved too difficult to overlook.

Which leads me into a recounting of one day in particular. We had only been in Rome for a couple of days when our group was given the chance to traverse the city without our faithful tour guide. This allowed for our group to buy a couple scoops of gelato each and eat it next to the elaborately carved sights of the Trevi Fountain. But one could only look at a slab of stone for so long before wanting to see the next hallmark feature. So, we wound our way through the labyrinth-like streets, taking time to enjoy the everyday sights and sounds of the modernized Renaissance city. After some time, we approached a stairwell that was adorned on all sides by overflowing locks of moss and ivy. The stairs themselves inclined at such a harsh angle that it required one to hold onto a side rail to avoid stumbling and falling to their death. We stopped there for a quick photo-op before panting our way on up to the top where it plateaued into an open stone courtyard. We all stopped to take a breath before turning our attention towards a gated building that was positioned next to our left.

There were a few other tourists huddling outside of the fence, all busy looking over maps of the city and wondering where to wander to next. And peculiarly, the door to the building behind them was left wide open, as if to welcome any other passersby who may be curious of its contents. Our teacher pointed us to the entrance's direction, and ushered us over in such a way that it felt as though we were intruding on someone's private property. Yet after walking through the doorway, a vault opened up and ran several meters high until it reached the peak of the ceiling. A confined entryway gave way to an environment that was locked into a historical time period that was unlike our own. And leading from it, past dozens of ornately laid stained glass windows, was a golden sarcophagus that sat in front of the pulpit.

Housed within the glass cube dangled a pair of steel shackles, a holy relic that is believed to be the very chains that bound the disciple Peter while he was under Roman captivity. The image was breathtaking, surely a spectacle that took away from yet another artifact in the chapel being a sculpture of Moses crafted by the infamous artist Michelangelo himself. Unbeknownst to us, we had waltzed right into the San Pietro basilica, a prized Church in the Italian Catholic scene. What captivated me the most about this sanctuary was just how much it contrasted from the rest of European artistry. While other pieces of architecture focused on the prominence and delivery of sophisticated art expression, this gem of a place slumbered peacefully behind a facade that appeared from the outside to be a simple hole-in-the-wall. But once you were inside, it transformed into a tapestry that was classic and timeless.

After spending an appropriate amount of time basking in the glory of the cathedral, we exited in file and returned to the still courtyard. Time was moving much faster than anticipated, and we were expected to regroup with our tour guide at a central location in the city. Just like that, we refocused on the significant trek ahead and put the ground beneath us. The trip moved forward, from neighbourhood to neighbourhood, from city to city. Soon, our understandably sluggish group was shambling down a plane boarding bridge at Heathrow, preparing for yet another lengthy flight that would take us home. Aside from the occasional snooze and subpar complimentary movie offered on the flight, my time was spent with eyes closed, playing back the experience like it was contained within a photo reel. So many elements of the pilgrimage had held significant value to me. For example, how could something surpass the adventure of riding atop the uppermost level of a passenger vessel as it slowly floats down the Seine waterway? No? Need it be more worthwhile? How about doing so while the lights of the Eiffel Tower shimmer at the moment the sun set? Now that is special! But still the reclusive little church in Rome kept coming back to my attention. And quite clearly, it became aware to me that it was less about what the site was and more about what it represented.

The demeanour of that worship space, despite its beautiful appearance, demanded respect. It called for the visitor to take a precious moment of their time, regardless of their background or understanding of religion, to live in intentional focus. The concept of respect had been one that I battled with for years.

Mainly because the term had been thrown around during familial disputes as a property that was expected of a child, as opposed to one that was earned. It was the crux of every argument that my parents used to defend themselves against behaviours that I deemed to be questionable or immoral. But I held firm in protecting my personal rights regarding civility. I was not a serf who merely pledged an irreversible oath to their lord's every command. Respect. It can't be offered if it is not returned in kind. This would be one of the many takeaways that I would hold close to my heart upon the return to my heartland.

With fingernail between the grip of an upper and lower tooth, a twisting motion of the hand began to tear the portions of keratin away from one another. The perforated nail struggled to cling onto the fleshy portion of the nail bed, until eventually, it tore up the right hand side of the finger and exposed a defenceless portion of raw skin. A shot of searing pain could be felt. It only took moments before blood began pouring out the open cavity. How could I do such a thing, once again? A band-aid was applied overtop of the carnage, which helped to match the other like minded appendages whose fates saw similar results not moments before. It was the reason why the family emergency kit was always depleted. Any time that something remotely worrying arose, the destructive habit would resurface. I considered whether or not this behaviour would appear less obvious if I simply curled my fingers into my fist so that others could not see them. It likely didn't matter. After the nails grew back, it was only a matter of time before history repeated itself.

SEAS OF YELLOW

CHAPTER NINE

AN EXTRAORDINARY, UNEXPLAINABLE DAY (FATE)

My high school years had passed by quickly, like those who had experienced theirs before me had warned. I graduated, parted ways with many of my peers, and began a fast transition of schooling at the University of Saskatchewan in the fall of 2014. It was difficult to gauge whether such a decision to start university (so early into post-grad life) was the right thing to do or not. The increasing attractiveness of the fabled gap-year had already laid claim to a variety of my fellow graduates. By early September of that year, my social media would be flooded with images of those travelling to locations such as Puerto Vallarta for all-inclusive vacations. For others, it was a local "stay-cation" where time was spent in the familiarity of Saskatoon. After metaphorically slapping myself back into consciousness, I would redirect my attention towards my long-term goal: the $50,000+ piece of paper from the post-secondary institution that implied I was smart and successful. It's easy to cringe at such a belief when one looks back at the trivial desires of their once immature mind.

That first year of university was a massive undertaking. I learned that writing essays was a lot more difficult than originally anticipated. Several of my paper submissions would return to me marked up with red corrective ink. The satisfaction within me from having completed them was tested against the constructive criticisms that their comments referred to. I also went through a messy, strange conclusion to a relationship with a girl I had met at church some six months prior. Looking back, our personalities would have never worked together long term. It may have very well been the best thing for the both of us to part ways. Nonetheless, I was resentful over how our relationship was handled, and I allowed my frustrations to fester for far longer than what was healthy. To top it all off, I had ruined my four-year plan to graduate with a Bachelor's Degree in Education because I had not acquired enough credits (I was just one measly course shy of the cut off) in my first semester. These factors were compounding on my mental health, and I was in dire need of some stability.

In an act of defeatism, I looked towards home, to those living there, to scavenge for morsels of support. Before going further, recognition must be given to my parents for showing initial interest in my academic pursuits. Mom was sitting beside me on the couch when I first opened my university acceptance letter, and watched as confetti paper flew out of the envelope and over the various nooks of the living room. Dad was the one sitting next to me the moment that course registration opened up online and, unfortunately, he witnessed several of my nervous breakdowns unfold as course enlistments closed within a mere matter of seconds. Without them in those moments, I would have likely lacked the sustainable drive in the adventure that was unfolding before me. But as I became more used to the expectations and responsibilities of post-secondary life, I began to note a shift in my parents' interests towards my experiences.

I remember many instances where I tried to bring up my burdens to my father, whom quickly dismissed said concerns because it surely "happens to everyone". It felt like a cheap shot to the realities of the situation(s). Other times, I would ask him for a second opinion towards a stance I took in an assignment. All I had been looking for was someone to comment on the clarity of my communication in the writing, to ensure that it didn't come across as unintelligible. He would refuse, stating that the content I was covering had "surpassed his understanding and ability" and would continue to do so as I requested a second or third time. A part of me now reflects on these circumstances wondering if I had genuinely wanted him to help me refine my writing abilities, or if I merely wanted to have him witness and engage in something that I was proud of.

If the first year of university was like that of gaining my sea legs, second year was where I had to batten down the hatches to avoid getting thrown overboard. Because of my mistake in allocating the incorrect classes per credit ratio the year prior, I had to make up for it by taking eleven courses in following academic year. Ridiculous is the only word that could describe those next eight months.

I do not remember much of this time, simply because I was so caught up in ensuring that my classes (and their requirements) were covered and that deadlines were being consistently met. The calendar that hung in my bedroom was designed with one purpose in mind, which was to keep the universe from imploding on itself. I became mesmerized by the ebb and flow of my weekly routine(s), which included the taxing bus rides that took me from *Avalon* to campus, and back again at the end of a long day of classes. I did not have much time to prioritize the maintenance of friendships (or so I thought), and often I would feel tinges of guilt strike at my heart when I became self-aware of how these decisions had ostracized myself from others. Certain friendships began to dissipate over time as a result. And although I had heard from people like Jonah from time to time, this recklessness had encouraged my brain to believe that spending time with him was a poor time management decision. Years later, I would ask him for forgiveness in this regard.

Despite the hectic schedule and overbearing responsibilities that I was facing on campus, I was thoroughly enjoying the content that I was learning. Anthropology, history, psychology, and archaeology were but a few of the subjects where I sponged up information that felt as if it were truly important and meaningful. As I sat alone in class, I could not be bothered with any of the problems that were occurring back at home. I could simply drown out the thoughts in my head with the droning of a professor's lecture. In fact, due to my schedule, I often left the house before anyone was awake and would return home as late as 10:00pm when everyone was preparing for, or were already, in bed. It was the perfect excuse to not see any of my family members. As I reflect on this thought, I would be lying to myself if I said that this type of attitude was not harmful to my perception of healthy relationships. I was taking an easy route by skirting around the problem; relishing in the moments of solitude and preferring to keep to myself for the sake of ease. When one thinks of a typical university experience, crippling isolation does not usually come to mind.

Things changed, however. Some may call it fate while others would call it divine intervention. Whatever it was, it would alter the course of my life (for the better) forever. One spring afternoon, I stood in the hall of the Arts and Science department, eagerly awaiting the previous class to vacate the room. I "needed" to secure a comfortable seat around the mid-central area of the learning space. A spot too close to the front was too vulnerable. Taking a spot at the back of the room made it easy pickings for the instructor to call out to me during class. Silly speculations, they were! The other students around me were doing the same; their facial expressions displaying a large spectrum of emotions ranging from grief to apathy. Everything about that day had appeared to be normal.

The door to the classroom eventually clicked open, and a flood of thankful students clawed their way out and into the hallway. They looked desperate for freedom. But just as I was about to enter the room, a familiar voice had called my name from further down the hall. As I paused to turn and see the source of the exclamation, I saw the friendly visage of a girl that I had graduated high school with. Bethany was her name. Her short stature was complimented by the jovial expression that was painted across her face. I had not seen her since graduation, and found it quite difficult to catch up given the brief amount of time I had to chat before class was to begin. In spite of that, it was nice to feel recognized in the disorderly environment.

Standing alongside Bethany was another girl, a stranger whom I had not recognized. She presented herself as the opposite of Bethany, as she was timid (in a peaceful manner). Beautiful shoulder-length brown hair flowed from her head. Even from the distance that I was standing from her, pockets of light freckles could be seen sitting atop her cheekbones. Her pursed smile and striking blue eyes pulled the entirety of her appearance together into one cohesive package. Noticing the awkward lack of attention in our conversation being directed towards this person, I turned and introduced myself to her. Her name was Tarah, and she just so happened to be enrolled in the same nursing program as Bethany and some other high school acquaintances of mine. Although short in duration, the introduction felt notably natural.

Class was set to begin, and I politely excused myself from the conversation with Bethany and Tarah in order to find a preferential remaining seat in the classroom. I proceeded to take out my various learning materials and anticipated the session to start. Upon wandering in, my professor introduced the topic of the day (was it language analysis or symbolic inferencing? Either way, it must have been boring enough to escape my memory) and began to teach. But as I attempted to listen to the instructor, my mind began to strangely shift in focus. I had become distracted by the events that had occurred in the hall just moments prior. I was captivated by the alluring young woman, Tarah, that I had just met. There was a tranquility surrounding the thought of her being. I attempted to snap myself out of this trance and focus once again on the class. I was, after all, paying an expensive fee for the lecture being provided. Shaking my head to expel the thought, I thought to myself, "How could I be so stupid to let innocent distractions impact my academic goal?"

"We need to scrutinize ... the importance of ... visual aids ..." the professor muttered on. Seconds had turned to minutes, and minutes had turned to hours. I could not believe it. I had let an entire class pass by without having any recollection on what was talked about or what was important to remember/study. Instead, I was thinking about Tarah. It was a baffling realization.

The rest of this tale played out in seamless fashion. The following month, I decided to do something that I never thought I would: directly reach out to a woman over social media and ask her out on a date. It is important to consider that Tarah was still a stranger to me. There was a genuine concern that perhaps I had read the original conversation of ours in a false manner. One thing was certain, if I didn't reach out to her somehow, I might never have the chance to come across a person who was as genuine or timely. So, I typed up a quick message on my laptop, and proceeded to stare at it with total uncertainty. I was petrified to hit the "send" button. I considered various hypotheticals, like her choosing to never reply to my greeting or even her responding with an explicit rejection. Closing my eyes and holding my breath, I reluctantly clicked the mousepad and listened to the subsequent "ping" that confirmed the transaction.

"Dear God, please don't let this be an oversight on my part," I thought. To my surprise, the computer chimed back shortly after. Tarah had responded to that message with warm reception. Her words provided me the same feelings of peace as those that were had in the campus hallway weeks prior.

Over the course of the following two years, our back and forth messages would transform into lengthy phone conversations. There were coffee dates (Tarah was an avid coffee drinker and bean connoisseur), walks down by the river, and impromptu road trips with no end goal in mind. And for once, the anxiousness that came with not having a plan ceased to be an issue for me. Her presence was enough to capture the entirety of my attention.

In 2017, we became engaged. By the summer of 2018, we were married. It was clear from the beginning that she was *the one*. This breathtaking woman was able to provide me with something that I had lacked throughout my entire life thus far: a sense of belonging. In fact, after spending copious amounts of time with her family, I had learned not only why she was poised in such a way, but I also realized just how socially butchered my own family was. Compared to my family's dynamics, Tarah's was kind, accepting, and ultimately, connected. I was dumbfounded by it all. Maybe I was even a little annoyed at just how much they loved each other. Remember, I could not stand being in the same room as my family for longer than an hour!

***

Without being aware of it, I had spent majority of my time outside of university classes at the condo where Tarah and her older brother lived. At first, I was uncertain about the tall, burly fellow whom Tarah called "Kris". However, upon later inspection, I realized that a kind and approachable man had existed behind the tall stature and woodsman beard that donned his being. She had loved him so much as to involve him in many of our earliest moments. Tarah recognized that I needed much more than a partner. She knew I needed a family. As a result, I had gained a brother.

It was here at the condo that the three of us would spend our evenings watching the *Edmonton Oilers* hockey games. Sometimes we would order pizza in, the bill quietly being paid by Tarah's brother without our knowing. Other nights, we would walk to the nearest fast-food restaurant and enjoy the conversations that accompanied our excursion. Whenever we needed a mental break from the challenges of post-secondary life, we would flick on a game system and play *Call of Duty* for hours on end. Never before had I felt such peace and clarity, specifically in regard to the people I wanted in my life. Noticeably absent was my desire to be back at home with my own flesh and blood. The condo was a sacred space to escape from all of one's problems.

I had never wanted to scare Tarah away because of the glaring realities of my familial situation, but at some point, I needed to be clear with her that my relationship with my parents was not to be considered "strong". I was afraid that my definition of the feelings pertained towards them would be misinterpreted as me being hostile or unwilling to adapt to their demands. How could I not be concerned? At the end of the day, I had grown up being told that my reactions to certain things was unjustified.

After mentioning and (unfortunately) witnessing a lot of these problems in person, Tarah's demeanour never faltered. Instead, she poured into me a fountain of empathy. On one hand, she was not shy to mention that what she saw wasn't healthy. She expressed how uncomfortable it was to sit in a room where people actively shouted at each other and got into each other's faces to do so. It was a valid concern. Regardless, she never blamed me for the ways that I felt about them. I had harboured an immense amount of shame in those earlier days. I was ashamed of who my family was and how they treated each other. Deep down, I was scared that I was going to (or already was) just like them. Tarah said otherwise. It was this mere acknowledgement alone that made me realize I was not just dating a good person; I was dating the person that I was destined to live the rest of my life with.

In my wedding vows, I recounted the day that I first met Tarah in that busy university hallway. I detailed the peculiar impact of our conversation and not being able to focus afterwards. That for some unexplainable reason, I had felt connected to her in ways that words could not express. I included how God had wanted us to find each other. At present, it is difficult to imagine a life without her. Our marriage is not flawless, as it follows the undulations of an imperfect reality. We are human. What changed between us first meeting each other and us living together was that we fought alongside in the same frontline. True to her heart, Tarah had never used any of these moments against me. And for that, I am eternally grateful.

The sanctity of special people and the relationships we share with them is something to never take for granted. We must do our best to give back to them. There are moments where I may feel like I am doing a disservice to Tarah, and ought to be trying harder in the shared moments of our life. Some situations appear small, like failing to clean up the dishes before she returns home from a night shift at work. Other situations appear more complicated, like those that elicit strong childhood sorrows and reactions. Pain seeps through the scar tissue. Events like communal family gatherings would often remind me of a life that I never had growing up. Yet, your people are right in front of your very eyes. The challenge is to speak up with them about these feelings, despite the nonsensical shame that one might be feeling. The people who truly care for you will stick around, and you for them.

"Look at all of these people," I tell myself. "There must be hundreds of them. All mingled about, with places to be and things to be done. I wonder what their stories are?" The cafeteria of the university was bustling with activity. Propped up top an elevated barstool, I watched as students followed the streamlined flow of movement from the terminal stairwell to the Arts and Science connection tunnel. Some were busy mid-conversation, and I could hear the audible rise and fall of their thoughts as they approached and departed from the counter where I was perched. Others appeared more closed-off, with their hoods pulled overtop their heads and noise being cancelled out by a pair of concealed headphones. Some wore the beautiful ornaments of their religion, like the hijab or kippah, while others wore next to nothing at all. It's a strange and eclectic environment.

I checked the time on my watch to make sure that I would not be late for my next class. With only ten minutes to spare, I packed up my belongings into my satchel and thrust myself into the flow of heavy foot traffic. And just like that, I was a part of the machine. I looked backwards to where I had just left, and my recently vacated seat was quickly snatched up by the nearest awaiting person. To be a piece in this chess match of life was fascinating. With every move, there was an expected subsequent reaction.

"What move do I make next?" I questioned.

CHAPTER TEN

ESCITALOPRAM

Nearing the end of my second year of post-secondary, I applied for admission into the *College of Education* at the U of S campus. This act alone served as a penultimate moment in my academic career. If my application was accepted, I could rest assured, knowing of the general trajectories that would take place in the following two years of study. If I was rejected, it was back to the drawing board. All that was holding me back was a scrutiny of my academic average and an inquiry with the references I had selected to speak on behalf of my personal and professional character. Curiously, it's as if I can still feel a break of sweat rolling down my forehead…

The strangest component of this process was awaiting a response from the screening board. So to avoid as much heightened apprehension over the whole ordeal, I would choose to ignore my intrusive thoughts that begged me to check my email inbox several times throughout the day. After losing to myself in this regard one afternoon, I got an answer.

"Welcome to the College of Education!" the subject line read. I let out a sigh of relief. Yet another assurance had been provided to me. I was going to become a teacher.

The following two years saw me undergo various cross-curricular studies associated with the practice of education. Such studies included politics and pedagogy, teaching and mental health, land-based education, etcetera. Sprinkled amongst such courses were fascinating engagement tactics used by the instructors. I recall one class in particular, focused on the art of teaching social studies/history to secondary students, utilizing crayons and paint materials for us adult students to engage with while we learned. Much of what was taught in these courses could appear as undisciplinary to some. Me? I loved the spontaneity of it all.

In the spring of 2018, I received my Bachelor of Education degree. I quickly entered into the workforce, and hungrily applied to the three nearest school divisions to serve as a substitute teacher. The demand for work was always present, and the opportunity to fill in for absent school teachers would allow me to begin creating a professional network, with long-term hopes of landing a job somewhere in or around Saskatoon. Thanks to my previous field experiences back in the College of Education, I had received several temporary teaching placements in both urban and rural settings. My first placement saw me in the rural community of Colonsay, a tiny farming town just a forty-six minute drive from Saskatoon. My second placement saw me across from *St. Paul's Hospital* at St. Mary's Health and Wellness Centre, an inner city school with a predominant Indigenous student population. Although very different from each other, both were eye-opening and fulfilling opportunities to hone my craft. The later opportunity to intern full-time at a school (for four months) saw me placed all the way out at Lloydminster Comprehensive High School. This institution peculiarly sat on the Saskatchewan-Alberta border, which forced me to travel and hunker down in the oil-patch city until the Christmas season began. It was equally informative as it was enjoyable. All of this to say, I had some experience to go off of when entering into the substitute teaching realm.

Many of my first substitute placements were located outside of Saskatoon, jumping to and from locations such as Duck Lake, Hanley, and Delisle. There was no direction on a compass where these contracts did not point! For example, one morning the dispatch crew of the rural school division offered me a full-day placement at a Hutterite colony, located in the RM of Lost River. Perhaps I should have taken the RM's title more seriously, for I had one heck of a time trying to locate the colony while aimlessly driving the gravel grid roads. Thankfully, I was able to wave down a local farmer that was driving his old, beat-down, Chevy pickup truck heading the opposite way. He chuckled at the encounter. It wasn't the first time someone tried to find the invisible community. Eventually, I was able to locate the tall structures of the colony that were sitting just on the horizon-line. I was met with the stone-cold stares of several men watching me pull into the front gates, but would later be eased of my nerves once the community welcomed me in with smiles and curiosity. It was a lovely day, and the children were naturally curious about this stranger that had come to teach them for a day. And I was curious about them as well. Teach in a two-classroom school in a unique cultural atmosphere? Check! Another bucket list item had been crossed off the list.

As the initial "honeymoon phase" of substitute teaching wore off, it became quite clear to me that this line of work was not for the faint of heart. Every waking hour of the day was spent attentively waiting for a phone call that would describe the type of work and location that you would be headed to for the day. One would feel an initial feeling of excitement in hearing a call, for a call meant that there was an opportunity to make some money. Yet, if the details of the assignment were unfavourable to one's credentials, the excitable emotions would swiftly turn to dread. On one occasion, I was to teach Kindergarten music theory for a full day's length. I remember a room full of five/six-year-olds striking away on xylophones, making the most abhorrently adorable sounds imaginable. I may not have been qualified for the job, but at least the kids appeared to be having fun!

Instead, it was the areas of High School humanities where I felt most at home. Contracts that included the subjects of history, english, and entry-level science were a welcome sight for sore eyes. However, the majority of calls that I had been receiving from dispatch were those offering work relating specifically to early elementary grades. A fair assumption for this reality may very well be that there were far more elementary institutions in the area than there were secondary. Another assumption, a likely one at that, was that I had been so eager to accept work at the start of my career, that an algorithm had picked up my recent accepted contracts and continued to tailor future job offers in similar fashion. Who knows? Speculation could only go so far as to wonder why this pattern continued to occur.

As I continued to work in the elementary realm, I began to note that my teaching experiences were becoming quite "hit and miss", as far as success was concerned. Some days, I had wonderful moments of teaching the assigned lesson plans and bonding with the students that I had met. Other days, the task of teaching was a living nightmare. Frequently I would show up to a school that I had never been to before and be presented with an incomplete (and in some cases, a lack of) lesson plan to work off of. My anxiety was simply unable to cope with the lack of structure or guidance on what I was supposed to do and achieve during the classroom teacher's absence. And so, utilizing the best of my abilities to shift and adapt instruction mid-lesson, I was able to scrape by many of these days with a semblance of success. With the handing in of the classroom set of keys to the school's front office, I was free to go. It was instant relief.

Amidst the turbulent teaching days, it was confusing to deconstruct the satisfied, yet disgruntled emotions I was feeling. The reality of it all was that another phone call would be coming in the near future. The thought of this began to terrify me to the point where, when my phone chimed with the ringtone of the dispatch service, I would enter into immediate psychological distress.

At this stage in our marriage, Tarah had acquired a nursing job in the small, rural town of Maidstone. Its terms were simple, yet broad; general admittance care by day and palliative care by night. On occasion, an ambulance would bring a unique case to the door, often involving a case of bodily injury caused by vehicle collision or something along the lines of a critical health event caused by the likes of stroke or heart attack. Due to its distance away from Saskatoon, it meant that Tarah would have to spend copious amounts of time away from myself and the basement suite that we were renting. And although I remained lonely at times during this stint, I was thankful that Tarah was able to stay at her childhood home with her mother and father in the nearby city of Lloydminster.

With my wife away from home, I had little to no supports in place to encourage me to pick up the phone whenever that foreboding ringtone shot through the speakers. Reluctantly, I would answer the call and listen to the automated voice list out the details of the given assignment. Upon hearing that the job was for somewhere located far away from the city, or in a school placement that I was frankly unqualified for, panic would set in. I would see myself react emotionally and physically to the lifeless robot speaking on the other end of the line. There were a series of months where upon getting ready for a workday, my stomach would churn in a volatile manner. My body would tell me that it would feel better if I simply vomited. And so, it became a routine to puke in the bathroom toilet before hopping into the car and driving off to the placement.

As time went on, my timidness with this way of work evolved to a point where I would refuse to pick up the chiming cell phone. Not only was I embarrassed of the display that I was showing to my wife, but I was embarrassed at myself for not taking a work call that was so desperately needed. As newlyweds, we had dreams beyond living in someone else's basement. We wanted to accumulate enough funds to cover a down payment on a house of our own. We wanted a home that was sizeable and safe enough for our future children to be raised in. Our current living conditions left much to be desired. We were located in an active crime area in the Western portion of the city, and the sirens of emergency vehicles began to permeate through to my memories and transport me back to the common scenes of my childhood.

One of the few saving grace's during this time (aside from the direct presence of my wife, of course) was when I received a dispatch call pointing me towards a school where I had already been and had good experiences at. Much of these placement requests were initiated by teachers whom left complete, engaging teaching materials for me to use in their absence. These calls were far and few between, sadly. I couldn't count on the consistency of multi-week contracts, and simply choosing the favourable job offers would mean days of inactivity work-wise. With such fluctuations so commonplace, I found the earlier confidence in my career path begin to wane. I gave myself a timeline for when I would give up this line of work and change my opinion on teaching as a whole. At the time, it would not have mattered if I had given up. If full-time teaching felt like an amplified version of substitute teaching, then why on Earth would I want to do it for the rest of my life?

Thankfully, I never had to commit to such a rash decision. In what appeared to be perfect timing, in regard to my mental health's breaking point, I was provided the opportunity to accept a teaching contract for a Grade 8 class placement in the city of Saskatoon. Although limited to one year, the decision was a no-brainer. Accepting the contract would mean that I no longer would have to deal with the misery that was substitute teaching. No more unknowns and no more changing expectations. Despite the development, I quickly realized that I had a lot of personal healing to do. The contract was a band-aid solution to a larger problem. The incidents of panic attacks and harmful self-reflection were becoming increasingly frequent, more so than ever before. Worst of all, my battle began to spill over into my marriage with Tarah. She began to notice that my anxieties were impacting the way that I responded to various situations. Even the slightest inconveniences in a day would set me off into a rage of frustration and self-loathing. If nothing were done, our marriage would have been irreversibly damaged forever.

It took years of convincing before I eventually acquired a doctor's appointment. Confirming the meeting was a huge first step, and walking through the door of the clinic was the second-most. Hesitancy coursed through my veins like an addict scoring a hit. It was tangible and unnerving. After I had signed in, I sat in a seat that was positioned in the far corner of the waiting area. Having my back to the wall felt comforting, as I was able to have a visible scope of anything that was happening around me.

"Levi?" the voice of the nurse called. Without saying a word, I stood up and followed the woman to an empty room located in the back corridors of the building.

"The doctor will be with you shortly," she stated. The door closed softly behind me. The room itself was virtually empty, filled with nothing but medical apparatuses, health pamphlets, and bottles of hand sanitizer. It was cold. It was quiet. As I sat there in silence, my mind became sentient, and began to attack itself. My pride had told me that I lost the battle, and that seeing a doctor meant that something was officially wrong with me. Humorously, it is apparent that my conscience was right about there being something wrong with me. I was just choosing to take that reality too personally.

The doctor would later knock on the door, introduce himself, and inquire about my reasons for coming into the clinic. He was a kind and soft-spoken young man, and there was never any air about his approach that implied an "otherness" about my circumstances. I described my symptoms to him in detail, ugliness and all. With a series of nods and verbal confirmations, he scratched down an approval for a prescription medication. The notepad read *Escitalopram*, a generic antidepressant. I was now diagnosed with *Generalized Anxiety Disorder* (GAD).

I began with a dosage that was low and purposeful in its design. It would be used to evaluate how receptive my body was to its presence and whether or not it could accurately target my symptoms. A skeptic at heart, I waited for some blatant sign to become known to me, one that would serve as undeniable proof that the medication was in fact doing what it was designed to achieve. The first few days of taking the small, white pill were highly pensive. After swallowing the foreign object and washing it down with a glass of tap water, I would sit upright on the living room couch and attempt to feel any form of change within my body. I can only imagine what my wife saw in me, as I glazily stared towards the wall, unmoving. It was impossible to detect if or when the medication kicked in. Perhaps my efforts were done out of desperation rather than skepticism.

Over the course of the following several weeks, the results of the medication began to grow more apparent. I went from puking in the bathroom each morning, taking two *Tums* tablets to quell the nausea, and internalizing my emotions to now having a more open, practical, and methodical approach to interacting with stress. One of the first "miracles" to occur during this time was my increasing ability to vocalize my feelings to others, specifically Tarah. I began to compartmentalize my stress triggers as contextual to the events in which they were created, and why an understanding of their origins was crucial to maintaining control over them. Logic and reasoning became important tools to curb a drifting mind. Little by little, I learned how to carry on with my days in a healthier fashion. I'd like to think that Tarah felt the same way, as generally, our moods and compatibility improved over time. It was my first dose of normal.

As time continued moving forward, the effectiveness of the original ten milligram prescription began to fade. Even though I had been warned of it doing so, I felt my anxious mind slip back into its familiar roots and try to convince me that I wasn't free from it quite yet. I was the *Pequod* sailing vessel, and my anxieties were *Moby Dick*. The two were inseparable. The thought of increasing my dose was largely intimidating. In complete transparency, I was still sparring with the interpretation of medication and its uses. Maybe it was the lack of money growing up that fuelled the "suck it up and deal with it" mentality that I often imposed upon my adult self. I also believe that I was living vicariously through a false belief that my body may know how to adjust to life without it. All I needed was a test drive to experience it. Maybe things would appear more recognizable moving forward? I could never have been more wrong.

My GAD symptoms began to return in full ferocity. Some even reappeared during the middle of teaching eighth grade school lessons. It was a clear signal that I could not remain stubborn and ignore what my symptoms were telling me. I went back to the doctor's office, tail tucked between my legs, and requested to have my dosage raised to twenty milligrams. To my medically inept mind, such an increase sounded enormous. Yet, the pattern continued the same way it had with my first prescription. My symptoms were calmed and the imbalance of my psyche began to level off. I could inhale positivity and exhale negativity.

My relationship with the concept of mental health took a huge turn during those fateful years. Undoubtedly, anxiety had gripped my ability to live what was considered a normal life. There were many moments where I would reflect on specific colleagues who worked in the same career field as me. These were the type of people who would comment on the ease of substitute teaching (even teaching in general). All I could do was seethe in private anger, for I was unable to tell them just how much the job had negatively controlled my life. In hindsight, I lacked vision in regard to what possibilities could be available to helping future students of my own who might struggle with similar conditions. Thankfully, I didn't pull the pin on my career choice. Eventually, I was able to see this vision turn into a reality.

I am certain that, at first, my perception on mental health was distorted by the types of language that I had heard people use in relation to it. In fact, upon sharing my recent medication acquisition with my own parents, I was given a blunt response:

"Well, everyone deals with stress Levi. It's not an uncommon problem". To them, my experiences were reduced to nothingness.

The reality of it all is that my mental health is best understood by me. Much like someone who undergoes a unique medical procedure, the surgery and subsequent recovery is a process that is distinctly felt by the individual. It is only within the past few decades that society has begun to validate the difficult nature of mental health conditions. Gone are the days of "tough love" and hiding one's skeletons in their closet. The opinions of others do not have any merit in regard to the length and path that one's healing journey takes. If you had asked me how people got through life, before I had started taking medication, I would have likely stated that determination alone could get the job done. I do not feel the same way now. The day that I sat in that doctor's office was a day of revelation. I had to swallow a massive pill (pun intended) of pride that kept me from getting the help I so desperately needed. Confusion, uncertainty, and fear are all things that come with healing. My newly-found understanding of this truth would later be one that would spearhead my personal philosophy on living life. As cliche as it sounds, it's okay to not be okay. Why does one's own self-esteem have to be dictated by another person? Frankly, it doesn't.

It was the year that the world stopped. While my students were away at their gym class, I had chosen to position myself behind my sturdy wooden desk in order to plan for the following day's teaching activities. It was a precious time not to be wasted. Rumours of a spreading contagion had been commonplace for months. Supposedly, the sickness had originated in China and was traversing the rest of the globe at a breakneck speed. And for the longest while, the topic was mere staff room squabble. It was limited to paranoiac speculations about how quickly it may reach the western world before the creation of a vaccine occurred. Meanwhile, hundreds (if not, thousands) were already dying in places such as Italy and the far East.

I continued to tap away at my work laptop until something out-of-place caught my attention on the monitor screen. From the bottom left-hand corner of the desktop, a tiny notification had popped up, displaying the words "Canada's Growing Health and Safety Measures". The face of the Prime Minister, Justin Trudeau, was plastered on the thumbnail. I felt compelled to click on the suggested media piece, despite not being one who was typically interested in political news coverages. My actions had caused a tab to open up on the CBC news site, and a video began to buffer before eventually tuning into a livestream.

Everything was shutting down. Restaurants, movie theatres, shopping malls, and the like were opting to put signs in their windows that turned their customers away. Masks began to appear as standard daily attire; turning from a tool originally used in medical circumstances to one of applied personal security. People also began to grow increasingly wary of their physical proximity to one another. They began to hug the walls of a room when it became too crowded and would dart glaringly towards someone who was unfortunate enough to mistakenly choke on air. The video that had remained playing through my computer emphasized and confirmed these realities. The face of the Canadian nation resolutely provided the first confirmed outbreak cases of COVID-19 in the country.

The following day, an email that was sent by my school's administration staff had confirmed the worst: all courses had been temporarily postponed and were to move online in the following two weeks. Just like that, and the entirety of the school year's momentum had ceased. As the face of the institution for my particular group of Grade 8 students, I stood in front of them that day and gave them the news I had been told. What resulted was a contorted mixture of celebration and horror. Behind my confident posture lied an uncertain apprehensiveness that made my feet feel numb. The students were then instructed to clear out their desks and lockers of all their personal belongings. The classroom bulletin boards were torn down without delay. Panicked parents arrived to the school within moments to pick up their child(ren) in a frenzied state. If this was the beginning of the apocalypse, it sure was reflective of commonly-held stereotypes and expectations.

From March of 2020 until April 2021, much of the prairie provinces remained locked down by federal and provincial mandates. The news continued to pour forth overtly negative statistics and projections regarding the virus' death toll and expected duration. Yet surprisingly, although modern societal foundations had collapsed at the start of the pandemic, alternatives were created for people to continue accessing the services that they once had. So, this naturally saw my teaching practices move from a physical classroom to an online platform. The navigating of a streaming service was challenging at first, but perhaps the more difficult element of the transition was the lack of recurrent students. Approximately ninety-percent of my pre-existing class attendance had disappeared following the initial closure of the school facility. Week after week, I would create custom content to help support those few remaining students who engaged with the platform I had maintained. The products of my work were definitely not pretty, especially those grim pre-recorded lectures that made me out to sound like an overly excitable individual. More-or-less, it was cringe-y to listen to. But if cringe meant that someone behind the computer screen was learning, then it was all worth it in the end.

To others dismay, I conveyed the taboo belief that the societal lockdown felt enjoyable. An introvert at heart, being able to work in the comfort of my home environment was something that I never took for granted. Waking up early to make a cup of hot chocolate, before checking my work emails whilst still dressed in my pyjamas, was bliss. Additionally, the pandemic had allowed for myself, like many others, to take a solid amount of time to review my personal understandings of the world. I questioned how it functioned and what role I played in it. This is not to say that acquiring a positive reading on a saliva swab had not dampened the mood. It reminded me of the reality of the situation, that what was happening outside of my home's doors was in-fact real. Going outside was a decision not to be taken lightly. But strangely enough, I could not be deterred. My anxious tendencies felt remarkably secure in the bubble of that basement suite, while the rest of the world continued to plunge deeper into disarray.

CHAPTER ELEVEN

FATHERHOOD

It was a lazy weekend afternoon, and I had been sprawled across the living room couch (scrolling through various pointless apps on my phone) when Tarah had called to me from upstairs.

"Levi! Can you come help me with something?" she asked. It seemed as though she had some kind of apprehension and urgency behind her request, yet, I ignorantly assumed that she was calling for me to have some small chore or task accomplished. So, I did what any dim-witted husband would: I prolonged my getting up and off of the couch and continued to lounge on the furniture. Keep this point in mind for future context.

Eventually, I did follow through on her beckoning and made my way up the stairs and to the master bedroom. Upon entering the room, my gaze was promptly directed towards our bed and the foreign mystery items that were placed upon it. Sitting neatly on the fabric of the duvet cover was an infant sleeper outfit, handwritten note with the words "Hello Daddy" sprawled across it in cursive lettering, as well as a positive pregnancy test. I was stunned. I placed my hands on the sides of my hips and stared blankly at the objects before me. Indeed, time had frozen and my consciousness had faltered. All the while, Tarah had been standing nearest the window in the room, not two feet away, smiling and eagerly awaiting my response. No words could have been able to express the emotions being felt in that moment. Perhaps it was even best to remain wordless.

I was in disbelief. All my life I had known that I wanted to be a father someday. It had seemed quite surreal that in that very moment, this dream had become a reality. I turned towards Tarah and we embraced each other with joy, excitement, as well as a pinch of uncertainty. Thankfully, my positive reaction to her surprise would mitigate most of the repercussions towards my tardiness in getting up the stairs.

We spent the following several months doing as any new parents would, preparing our newly acquired home with all of the furnishings required to welcome and raise a child. Tarah, being the instinctual and intelligent maternal figure she is, began to construct a list of essentials that would be needed before the baby arrived in the spring of 2021. One of the spare rooms that had been previously used for storage was cleared out and redesigned into a nursery. Various weekends were spent perusing malls and outlets for assorted parenting equipment. Who knew there could be so many different forms (and price ranges) of car seats!

To lighten the burden, Tarah and I had created a baby gift registry to make it simpler for our friends and family to support our growing needs. We were greatly humbled as packages began to arrive at our doorstep from people of all kinds and personal histories. It wasn't until these gifts were brought into the newly-curated nursery that a second dose of reality was administered. Yet, as Tarah busily prepared, I found myself sitting back and pondering what more I could do to become invested in the arrival of our firstborn. I was not as educated in this life transition as she was. She was a labour and maternity nurse, at this point, after all. I was a middle school teacher, which meant that my targeted youth experience was focused on the years that fell well after the newborn stage. So what could I practically do to welcome this child?

By the time that the Christmas season had rolled around, which was a mere matter of months away from our April 4th due date, I had returned home from work for the weeklong holiday. Of course, I had brought home a flurry of objectives to be completed before returning back to the office. Essays were to be marked, lessons needed to be planned, and it seemed as though there would not be enough time to complete everything on my to-do-list. Thankfully, the weeklong break allowed for some extra "wiggle room" to help mitigate the symptoms of my anxiety. The added weight of familial gatherings (on top of work deadlines) created an intimidating foe.

It wasn't until there was a brief pause in the midst of that week where I had thought about the state of the nursery room upstairs. Sure, a crib had been purchased and assembled, as well as a dresser for the increasing counts of little clothes, but the room remained rather generic and simple. It lacked a "wow" factor, so to speak. Tarah and I had been contemplating the theme of our child's room for quite some time, and upon finding out the sex of our son (an exciting and surreal experience at that), we decided to theme it on the North American plains. His little room was quickly endowed with related aesthetics that pulled all of the fundamentals together into one cohesive unit. With how much time Tarah spent in the room, I could tell that she was happy with our progress. I, on the other hand, still felt an absence in the final product. And so, Tarah and I discussed what I could do to add a personal touch to the room. We eventually agreed that I would attempt to paint a mural that would be hung overtop of the crib. We agreed to the image of a buffalo.

Now, it's important to state that I am no natural artist. My mother had honed such talents, and I could only hope that some of that genetic code would be passed on to me. For her, art was effortless. A seemingly unprovoked stroke of graphite or smear of acrylic. And the closer that this project's execution date neared, the more I became nervous if I was going to be able to pull it off. Together, Tarah and I spent copious amounts of time scanning the internet for reference images to assist in the creative process. The more we searched, the more my apprehensiveness grew. But despite my fears, Tarah's calm and reassuring attitude helped reinforce a belief in myself that I could accomplish this task.

An assortment of coloured paints was bought alongside a large, white poster board. The time to create was officially underway. Throughout the following three hours, I meticulously brushed the poster board and shaped the image into the likeness of a bison. It is strange to reflect upon the experience in retrospect, because I had become so hyper focused on the task that it is remarkably difficult to pinpoint my exact emotions as the image was being produced. Nevertheless, the final product had turned out uniquely well. Perhaps the painting would never stand up to the skill and detail present in other professional works. However, I had finally acquired a sense of fulfillment in knowing, that in some discrete and small way, that I had done something for my boy. He would be able to sleep in his own little bed underneath the careful watch of the painted buffalo.

When I had first laid eyes on that positive pregnancy test, I was filled with anticipation. I was going to be a father! However, a very real concern came to mind when I had more time to consider what that actually meant. Due to my difficult, and oftentimes traumatic, experiences with parents and child-rearing practices as a youth, I began to harbour significant doubt towards my own ability to raise a child with love and humility. I had grown up in an environment where screaming at your children for doing something wrong was a completely justified act. I had been mocked for the way that I responded to provocations that spurred my anxious mind. I had been manipulated into thinking that those ways of parenting were standard. These fears had become actualized over the many years that I had dated and been married to Tarah. Rather embarrassing family dinners would occur at my parents' house where derogatory comments would be directed toward someone, and a retaliation would ensue. Tarah was often able to witness times where my parents made questionable decisions in regard to familial matters. Unbeknownst to her, for I had not been particularly vocal about my feelings with these matters, I worried that I was but a product of my parents' decision-making, and that I was destined to become just as much of a failure as them. In time, there were moments where I would contrast my own behaviour against what I had experienced growing up. I analyzed whether or not I had seen this conduct from my mother or father. I was in a constant state of confusion about my changing identity.

On April 2nd of 2021, we welcomed Milo into the world. Despite the feeling as though we were waiting for an eternity for him to arrive, it was shocking just how sudden he was there in the hospital room with us. I fondly remember his first moments with much clarity and imagery. After being delivered, Milo was quickly placed onto his mother's chest, and he began to wail a sweet cry that demanded more comfort be provided to him. I remember his mother's serene face, smiling and looking down on the perfect creation that she had made. I remember that this was one of the only moments in my life where I cried tears that felt genuinely good to let go of.

We still had to adjust, like any parents do, to this new phase of life. There were many nights where Milo would cry for his mom or seek the security of his father's warmth. There were days where Milo struggled to defecate, causing him extreme discomfort in his juvenile digestive system. Those times were difficult, and wife and husband turned to one another for support and reassurance. Regardless, they are treasured moments that one wishes could be bottled up and taken with wherever they go.

As Milo began to reach milestones and display certain developmental goals, I began to veer further away from the notion that I was destined to be failure of a parent. It wasn't my ability to change his diapers that proved myself wrong. God knows how much more of a mess I made than his mother at that job. It also wasn't my ability to prepare a bottle of formula. It was the smile that my son gave me in those earliest moments that told me that he loved me, and that he did not care about a past of mine that even he was unaware of. It was in those moments that I made an intentional decision to put a barrier between what had happened to me and what I was going to do about it. I had (have) the ability to be the kind of father that I wanted to be.

None of this transformational change in thought would have been possible if it were not for my wife and son, whose views of me remained unchanged throughout those early moments of our shared lives. Fast forward a couple more years, and this truth was once again reinforced with the welcoming of our second son, Denny, to our family. This goes to show that life is what you make of it, and who you hold close. Your psyche has the potential to either control or alter your world. Peace is a choice.

Children are precarious creatures. Spontaneous at times and ritualistic at others, it is fascinating to watch the inner workings of their cognition function from behind their expressive little faces. In our house, the night time routine was well scripted, so to administer a slow, calm transition into a time of deep sleep. Following dinner, one of us parents would fill a bathtub with warm water, soap, and toys, and subsequently plop Milo into the growing mountain of suds. He would spend copious amounts of time frolicking about, spilling water overtop the sides of the tub and laughing away at the mishap. And although it took some convincing, he would eventually be pulled out and wrapped into a pre-warmed towel that was tightened around his body like that of a maximum facility straight-jacket. Next, it was time to put on pyjamas. This is where the art of distraction came in handy, as conversations surrounding the day's activities would be had while a set of pants and shirt were sneakily maneuvered onto his sprawling limbs.

"Alright buddy, come rock with Papa on the rocking chair," I would whisper as I lifted the tiring boy up and into my arms. Once in the confines of the chair, a book would be cracked open, and the sighs of a pre-slumbering child would begin to echo. I don't have memories of this kind from my childhood. No matter how hard I try to reach for them, nothing rings clear. Is this why I have become so hyper focused on familial matters? Maybe I can create moments for my children to remember by the time they are my age?

Stop it! Stop overanalyzing! Focus on the here and now. Feel the warmth of the napping child on your lap, and the rising breaths of their chest. Take it in and turn your brain off.

And just like that, I am snapped back into reality. I stretch my eyes open, roll my neck around, and scan the room from left to right. The light shining from outside the window indicates that it is still evening, and that Milo should be put to bed. As I position him in such a way to carry him effectively, he momentarily shudders awake and wraps his arms around me.

"The Star Wars book, Papa? We finish[ed] it?" he asks.

"Yup, we finished it bud. It's time to go to sleep," I respond. Without giving it much thought, I respond to him once more, not sure of the expected reaction. "May the force be with you, Milo". I then kiss his head atop his curly, blonde hair. He shuffles some and lets out yet another comforting sigh.

"May the force be with you, papa". His sweet voice replies just before he buries his face into the nook of my neck. All this time had intended to be was just a moment to read books. What it turned out to be was a moment of wholesome bonding and healing. Maybe I'm doing something right. I hope I am.

CHAPTER TWELVE
"I'M BLEEDING"

Several years go by, and I find myself becoming increasingly acquainted with the levelling phase of my mid-twenties. What originally began as a temporary grade eight teaching contract transitioned into a continuous high school teaching position, where I was to teach an array of courses ranging in subjects from history, to english, and even photography. This shift in teaching focus, despite causing notable changes in its preparation and delivery, proved to be the perfect affirmation I needed to convince myself that my efforts in the community were not going unnoticed. So, I continued to dig deep into my work, letting the responsibilities of my career sustain my concentration and need for assurance.

Another marker of life's changing pace was Tarah's and my

purchasing of a down payment on a new home. Much of our early years of marriage were spent carefully budgeting for such a financial hurdle, yet the process of searching for a home was starkly spontaneous. After walking through a couple of open houses, the two of us quickly noted various features that we liked, and others we did not. At this point, we were still childless, but knew that we would start trying for kids soon. It just so happened that on a day where the intent was never to pull the trigger, so to speak, we ended up aggressively offering a price on a two-story new build. The house had not even been listed on the market yet, but there was something urging us to have our realtor pull some strings. Our interest proved beneficial, and our offer was quickly accepted.

What more could we have asked for? In fact, we were greatly humbled by the puzzle pieces of life falling perfectly into place. All that was left was to sit back and enjoy breaking in our new home with the comforts of our belongings.

***

It was Valentine's Day, 2023. The school bell had just rung, indicating that the students had a mere five minutes to make it for attendance for their first period class. Sitting at my desk, I hovered overtop my teacher planner, scanning the lesson plans I had created just the day before. Judging by what the notebook had written on it, it was to be a fairly exhaustive day consisting of formal lectures and time-consuming learning activities. No matter, for these types of teaching days happened from time to time. It was bound to at least provide some form of engaging responsibility on my end.

The overhead speaker chimed, and students in my classroom rose from their desks and ceased their conversations with one another. The national anthem played first, and was followed by *The Lord's*

Prayer.

"For thine is the kingdom, the power and the glory, forever and ever. Amen". And with that, the day was set to officially begin. I took a deep breath in, released, and pointed my attention back towards the task at hand. I cracked a couple of jokes to the class about it being February 14th, for it was an obvious area of agonizing conversation for a group of teenagers. To me, they were adorable in their awkwardness. To them, I was a product of aging, merely a man making jokes about a topic that they were far more familiar with than I. Humour aside, the rise I was able to get out of them set the tone for the morning. It was bound to be a good day.

That was when my phone chimed from within my pants pocket. Not thinking much about it, I allowed the notification to pass by without so much as a mental note. Surely I would find time within the next hour to see who was messaging me. When the opportunity arose, I flashed the face of the phone my way and was met with a short text message.

"I'm bleeding". It was Tarah. Instantly, my face went flush, and I leaned onto the nearby corner of my desk to stabilize myself. The previous thoughts in my head evaporated and swirled noxiously. Somehow I was able to paw my way through a response text, asking her to describe how bad the bleeding was. My fears had been actualized when she confirmed that it was steady. I scanned my room of students, most of which were independently working on a task I had provided them with. They didn't know. They couldn't see past my facade. As I slowly ambled my way around their work stations, the occasional student would inquire about a particular challenge in their learning. The memory of my responses are hazy. In the moment, I wasn't engaged with them. Instead, I was looking at the world around me from within the imprisonment of my skull. I was hearing noises at a distance, and a fuzzy sensation could be felt winding its way around the fingers on my hands.

The bell chimed once more, which roused the students from their seats and ushered them into a frenzy of movement. I gave a faint-hearted smile to those few students who locked eyes with mine as they exited the room. I then slumped into my office chair and placed my face into the palm of my right hand. It was then that I just sat there, in complete silence. This wasn't supposed to happen to people like us. We had done everything to avoid this kind of problem. Did God hate me? Further verification of Tarah's condition would prove that she was, in fact, having a miscarriage.

We had only known about this pregnancy for around two weeks before the miscarriage occurred. It may not have been long, but we were swept up in the joy of having another child. While I was busy at work, Tarah was out shopping for newborn clothes. When I got home after a day away, we would exchange possible baby names that interested us. And perhaps the most powerful confirmation of all, we told Milo that he was going to be a big brother. His smile said it all. He was ready for that.

The first thing I did when I learned of the terrible fact was turn to my teacher planner. At the top of the page, beside the date, I impulsively wrote in red ink "I love you, my child". It was as if someone was playing a cruel joke on us, on a day that represented love of all days. I stared at the drying ink, noting its changing potency the longer I remained affixed to it. I considered whether or not I should go directly home. I didn't have a strong enough plan to leave for an emergency substitute filling, and so I opted to see if I could make it to the end of the day, which I thankfully did. My stubbornness had prevailed once again.

Tarah's emotions fluctuated throughout the day, understandably so. The few messages throughout the remainder of that day told me everything that I needed to know. She was struggling. So much so that she drove to the school and waited in the parking lot for me to be released of my duties at the end of the day. I can only imagine what she saw, as my defeated figure made its way towards the car. I knew that I had to be strong for her, but it required a level of strength that seemed so difficult to grasp. All that needed to happen was for us to embrace one another. The moment I got in the car, she wrapped her arms around my neck and lodged her face into it. The gasps of air that shot in-between her sobs resonated deep from within the vehicle. We didn't say anything to one another for what must have been ten minutes. We then proceeded to phone our family doctor and provide her with an update as to what had happened.

The subsequent days were arguably more burdensome than the day we lost our child. While I internalized most of my frustration, Tarah's was thrust forth in the form of unpredictable mood swings. It was common to wake up in the middle of the night and to hear Tarah crying into her pillow. The instant I rolled over to console her, her symptoms grew more intense. On a different occasion, Tarah was upstairs in the master bedroom having a conversation with her mother who was gracious enough to sacrifice her time to stay with us shortly after the incident. As the two of them talked, the tone and reality of the situation grew increasingly apparent, as it did in regular intervals for my poor wife. Tarah then shrieked an anguished cry of desperate attention. I had been sitting downstairs on the couch with Milo, watching children's cartoons, when it had happened. The sound caused me to sprint up the stairs and into the on-suite bathroom, only for me to find her sitting with her back against the tub, in an obvious state of hurt. It was obvious that healing was going to require a lot of time.

Eventually, we were able to talk more openly about our loss without evoking similar reactions. This did not mean that our wounds were healed over. If truth be told, they were just beginning to scab. We stopped buying children's apparel (most of the pre-bought stuff was given away to others whom we knew were expecting) and we avoided talking to Milo about his, now lost, sibling.

In order to move forward, Tarah and I needed to gravitate towards each other. And we did. Although it may come across as sounding odd, other than the times where I witnessed Tarah during labour, these specific weeks mark a time where I saw her display innate resiliency. She fought like an animal that was backed into a corner and had nothing to lose, and she still won. For all I know, I may have been distracted from this fact at the time. My career-focused mindset had kept me clear from seeing her strength on full display. The onus is on me, for that.

Now that moment remains an important marker on our relationship timeline. It happened, and there's nothing that we can do to change that. However, how we reflect on that terrible day is a choice. So let this be a comment on the state of affairs regarding marriage. Never lose sight of your spouse. You are obligated to see them for their weaknesses, talents, and their journey. I love you, my wife.

As we pulled into the entrance of the village, I noted how much the "Welcome to Mistusinne" sign had aged since the last I saw it. It was yellowed, cracked, and warped.

"Somebody ought to fix that," I thought. I even knew where the paint cans sat in the workshop. The fix would only take a mere matter of minutes.

The visit began as most in the past had, by circling the three loops of the community and seeing if anything had changed. One lot, whose previous architectural occupancy had burned down several years prior, still sat empty and charred. The local playground had favoured from a couple of upgrades, a far cry from the classic wood and rubber structures that donned the space in my childhood. Other than that, there was a tangible hint in the air that felt notably untouched.

It had been two years since I had been to Lake Diefenbaker. A sizeable argument had occurred between Tarah and I and my mother and father, again. The collateral of this fight saw my set of cabin keys "borrowed" to my younger brother, Liam, never to be returned again. It was clear to us that Mom and Dad were using this profound place to make a statement about their displeasure of our standing up for ourselves. I hurt for the longest time, as a result. There was a possibility that I may never be able to give my own children an opportunity to experience the lake like I had growing up. All that was within me wanted to confront my parents about their vile approach at retribution. It felt like a low blow, intended to cause long-lasting pain. But I couldn't follow through on such goaded desires. And so, I took several steps back. If what they wanted was a reaction, then they weren't going to get one.

"Papa, we['re] here?" Milo squeaked from the back of the car. His eyes were focused on the passing features outside of his unrolled passenger window. His tufts of golden hair were flapping wildly atop his head.

"We're here, Milo! Should we go see the water?" his mom and I replied. He quickly agreed to the offer, and our car turned onto the single lane gravel road that led towards the village's boat launch. As we took a final corner past the wild, overgrown prairie grasses, an expansive view of the lake opened up. The wind then picked up even more than before; the expanse of the water's surface acting as a highway for the gusts to speed across. We parked the car near the top of the launch ramp and unloaded Milo from the car so that he could stretch his legs. The second his toes hit the sand, he took off towards the shoreline. I couldn't help but smile at the little boy running and laughing without a care in the world. He looked so happy.

It was then that a guttural punch of reality hit me in the stomach. I was reminded of why our short visit to Mistusinne looked the way it did. There was no walking up the cabin steps and rediscovering the long lost friend. We wouldn't be able to spend the night there, as my grandfather (who built the lodging), had intended it. Tarah slowly walked up to me and wrapped her arms around my waist.

"Happy Father's Day," her voice rang soft and sweet. Her touch alleviated some of the pain that panged in my heart.

"Thank you, dear," I returned, locking hands with hers. The wind continued to blow sand up and over the top of the bluffs and right into the base of our heels. It caused a pin-prick sensation that would make one laugh and wince at the same time. The clouds overhead rolled swiftly against one another, at times blocking out the light of the sun and creating a spellbinding pattern of shifting shadow-work across the length of the shoreline.

"Chase me, Papa! Chase me!" Milo cried out. I did, to his delight. It was scenic, this perfect moment in time.

When we had enough of the onslaught of blowing sand, we made our way back up the ramp and into the safety of the vehicle. It shook violently as everyone secured their seatbelts and brushed off their feet. And before putting the car into "drive", I placed my hands upon the steering wheel and stared out across the body of water. My mind became overwhelmed with visions of the past. Not a few years earlier, I stood in this same spot, alone, taking in the sights of the valley with reverence and admiration. I'm certain my eyes glazed over, as they usually do when I become transfixed on a thought for too long. Tarah placed her hand on my thigh, instantly snapping me back into consciousness.

"I'm good. I am." I tell her. That was but a fraction of the truth. I felt as though I was losing connection to this place. It felt unfamiliar, but familiar all the same. A confusing concoction of twisted memories alongside modern influences. I then put the car into gear and drove back towards the village entrance. We left as soon as we had arrived.

SEAS OF YELLOW

CHAPTER THiRTEEN

CONVERSATIONS WITH A SAINT (EMDR THERAPY)

"What does your box look like?" the therapist asks, her eyes carefully scanning the way that the strange question impacts me. I unintentionally flinched upon hearing the request.

"Pardon me?" I respond. I begin to dart my eyes around the room, looking for a physical box that she may have been referring to. Maybe my consciousness lapsed when she asked me originally.

"I know it might sound weird, but I want you to visualize a fictional space where you can place your negative thoughts. Everybody's box is different". She places her hands neatly upon her lap and once again awaits my response.

"Is it okay if I close my eyes?" I ask. The task begged for further concentration and an elimination of any possible distraction.

"Of course," she confirmed. My eyelids shut, and after a few seconds of silence, an image began to appear from within the confines of darkness.

"The box is moderately sized, probably 2x2 feet. It's made of … stainless steel that has been brushed down with steel wool".

"Good. What does the lid of the box look like?" the therapist inquired.

"It's also stainless steel. The molds of the top fit perfectly atop the base. It's … simple". I was entranced in the process of illustrating this fabricated material.

"And how does your box close? Is it secured? Or is it easy to open it?" she continued. I laughed, not because of the seeming absurdity of the activity, but because of how it was becoming increasingly simple to let my mind illustrate the details of my box.

"There are four steel prongs underneath the edges of the base of the lid. When it is placed on the base of the box, they secure by sliding into it. It's durable. It can't be broken into easily".

"Ah! I see. It sounds like your box is made to contain some pretty tough things". Her consistent commentary continued to provoke in me an acute understanding of the design of the object.

"Yeah" I reply. And for a second or two, I sat in another period of silence, the image of the contraption slowly spinning in front of me.

"You can open your eyes now". Upon following the appeal, I slowly became reacquainted with the familiar sights, sounds, and smells of the room. I could once again feel the texture of the cozy rug underneath the soles of my feet. I also saw a whiteboard on the far side of the wall that had various "motivational" messages written on it, intended to be used in conjunction with some other persons healing process. A portion of sunlight was peeking through the corner most windows, providing a sense of warmth and comfort. Blinking helped ease and quicken my recalibration. The therapist, once noting my renewed concentration, pressed on.

"This practice can be used the next time that you feel yourself 'slipping'. Take a moment to step away, to slow down, and imagine yourself placing your worries in that box you created. What did you feel when you opened your eyes for me?"

"I felt ... peaceful," I acknowledged. It was true. I had been effectively grounded, and nothing outside of that therapy room was moving at the same pace that it had before.

***

The journey to attain professional help was unsteady. On one occasion, Tarah and I hurriedly rushed to get showered, dressed, and in the car to make it in time for an appointment that was scheduled for early morning. Our patience for one another had been tested in the events of those preparations, and by the time that I sat in the driver's seat and closed the door of our car, the blood within my body had boiled and my muscles were contracting. Breathing intensified to a point where it became laborious. It was just me left alone with my thoughts until Tarah popped open the passenger door and sat in the adjacent seat. We were ready to go. Nothing was said, not for a while that is. My foot pressed harder on the pedal than usual, maybe as a semi-conscious effort to get to the appointment sooner. Gauging my wife's body language, it had obviously caused her some discomfort. It was upon pulling onto the freeway exit ramp that the events of the morning escalated into a dramatic finale. An oncoming truck poised itself in the left bound lane. I glanced at my driver's side mirror, evaluating the distance between our two vehicles. It was closing in on us, and someone was going to have to adjust. Judging by the truck's apathetic change in speed, it appeared as though I was being told to adapt. With this, I snapped and punched my boot on the accelerator, sending our SUV into a lurching surge forward. The engine roared and I swung the tail of the car in-front of the nose of the opposing truck.

"Levi, stop!" Tarah stated with a profound blend of stern protection. It was enough of a reaction for me to become aware that I was quickly losing control, and her voice subsequently caused tears to pour down the sides of my face. I had reached my breaking point.

"I think it's time to get you some help," she followed.

It was within a matter of weeks afterward that I reached out to a local therapist to acquire help. And in that initial stride to reach for it, a wave of complex emotions began to swell from within me. At first, I was met with my own severe defeatist attitude. I told myself that I had lost my battle. I was supposed to beat the odds and get through these emotions on my own accord. Next, I felt guilt for not accepting defeat sooner. How long did I prolong (and worsen) the state of my mental health because I had been so stubborn? Lastly, and worse still, I lamented on the impact that my mental health had on my family. Although intense, those first moments of sitting down across from a professional proved to be a monumental turning point in humanizing these emotions.

***

The conversations with my therapist continued in the months and years to come. Some sessions proved more difficult than others, due to the ever-changing severity of my symptoms. Remember, so much of it was caused by external forces as much as internal. Most sessions began with a catch-up period, where I filled her in on the events that had happened since our previous meeting that caused me concern. It was her way of learning more about me and the elements of life that had their strongest grip on my efficacy.

An area of increasing potency was that of my relationship with my parents. Eventually, she identified the tarnished relationship as being one of core prevalence to my anxiety. It came as no surprise to either of us. I had imparted many disturbing stories to her regarding the ways that my parents had reinforced expectations through manipulation and blackmailing. Not to mention, my challenged ability to communicate these confused feelings was likely a result of narcissistic parenting.

"Am I crazy?" I would ask her after dispelling a vat of emotional baggage into the room. "I'm serious. If there is anything that I have or will say that comes across as completely backwards, you need to tell me that I'm in the wrong. I need to know that my thoughts are valid". With eyes locked on mine, her posture leaning into that of my own, she told me that I was human. She mentioned that what I was feeling was a natural response to my brain's strife. I breathed a sigh of relief. The thoughts had not immediately disappeared, but at least they had been temporarily tamed.

***

"What is it that you want people to know?" she would later ask.

"I don't know, that's an interesting question," I would ponder. "I suppose I want people to know my authentic self. None of the made-up stuff that others like my parents had others believe. I want them to know the truth. They should know what happened behind closed doors." I paused, unable to continue my train of thought.

"I'm sorry," I apologized, not knowing what had come between my thoughts and the words struggling to escape from my mouth.

"You know, in this session alone, you have sought apology several times. Do you know what that tells me?" the therapist urged. I shrugged my shoulders, avoiding eye contact from embarrassment. "It's a sign of trauma. You likely aren't even aware of yourself doing it".

"I'm sorry, er…" I caught myself before saying any more. We both laughed at the irony. Then the weight of her observation sunk in.

***

The cycle of returning for help while bringing with me new afflictions became routine. It was exhausting. The relationship with my parents continued to remain stagnant, and in some cases, worsened. I felt conflicted about being in contact with them. They were my parents after all, and it should feel normal to want to maintain a bond with them. However, after many in-person disputes and over-the-phone yelling matches, enough was enough.

One argument stands out in particular. One day, my father decided to phone me late in the evening. I had been in the act of getting Milo down to bed when my ringtone cried out. I reluctantly answered the call and passed Milo off to Tarah so that I could talk in privacy. I had anticipated my father to comment on a previous decision of Tarah and I to spend some time without contact from them. It was a measure on our end to protect our son from the collateral damage of our quarrels. He was just over one-year of age, and we deemed it unnecessary to have him within earshot of a conflict that had profound consequences to it. It wasn't long into our talk when my father's tone shifted and his voice turned stern (even derogatory). He began to interrogate my approach to solving the issue, claiming that I was meddling with the relationship that they were to have with their grandson. Up until that point, I had held composure. I wanted to listen to him intently and identify the areas of our relationship that could be mutually restored. However, all that came through the phone speaker was a list of complaints and ill-stated claims. And so, my composure broke. I snapped at Dad harshly, calling him out on his inability to empathize with my feelings. The phone call ended in bitterness. And from that moment forward, I knew that things would be different.

"I think I need them out of my life". The words hurt as they crawled up and out of my vocal chords. "I know that it is a serious decision to make. I just don't think I can do this anymore. They can do this to me. I can take the brunt of their attacks. But I cannot have them target my wife and son". I looked to my therapist for advice and I was met with affirmation.

"There will be sacrifice involved in a decision such as this. But you know what needs to be done to support your family, Levi. You do". That day, I was taught that I had been looking at the concept of boundaries all wrong. Rather than be viewed as antagonistic and retaliatory, I needed to view them as necessary. Boundaries are important features that help foster healthy relationships, regardless of whether the relationship is cordial or not.

***

Two years go by and my small family and I find ourselves estranged from my parents. For the first time in my life, I decided to truly stand up for myself and what I believed in. Tarah and I cut off communication with Mom and Dad and stated our reasons for doing so, in effort to provide them with some transparency. It went how anyone would expect. We were met with an onslaught of victimizations.

The most curious result of this decision? My small family and I were able to experience some of the most peaceful years we had ever had together. There was no more interrupting of bed time routines, nor were there any uncomfortable family gatherings. But like before, the trade-off saw me deal with several invasive doubts regarding my loyalty to family. It's a curious thing that such reflections can happen all the while one is actively avoiding that very kind of betrayal. Thankfully, I had the right supports in place to keep my mind at bay. Firstly, there's my wife: the woman who vowed at the pulpit to support and love me in both life and death. She must have taken that promise seriously, as she could have ran at the first sign of trouble. And boy, was there a lot of it. Then there's my children. The smiles they give when I walk in the front door say what a million words cannot. Then there's people, like my therapist, who selflessly offers her time to sit and listen to me unpack the miseries of a 27-year old's childhood chest of emotional wounds. I'm convinced it's the practice of sainthood.

The way forward is paved with uncertainty. But I found help to curb the apprehension. Over time, talking to my therapist became an easier thing to do. Our relationship grew out of trust and respect, and as a result, we were able to reach deep within the archives of my memory and pinpoint the origins of my psychological damage.

"Look at my fingers and don't let them sway" she stated. Her hand moved in the makeshift shape of a crucifix and other rhythmic patterns before being lowered back to its beginning position. I humorously called her out on the practice of voodoo and hypnotism, which made me feel slightly more comfortable with the foreign tasks she had given to me. I'm certain that she was well aware that the skeptic in me was beginning to accept that seeking help was the right thing to do.

---≋---

"*Adopt responsibility for your own well-being, try to put your family together, try to serve your community, try to seek for eternal truth... That's the sort of thing that can ground you in your life, enough so that you can withstand the difficulty of life*".

– Dr. Jordan B. Peterson

CHAPTER FOURTEEN

LORD, I NEED YOU

For starters, I wouldn't consider myself to be the "raise your hands and holler" type of Christian. Much of this is likely due to my conservative, Reformed upbringing. However, I would be in denial if I had never considered tapping into the unfamiliar practices of other denominations, should it mean that God could make himself feel more present during the tough times in my life. But this isn't a conversation about which theology is the most authentic to a disciple-like practice. No, it is more a reflection on my own grappling with the concept of a God who remains so tantalizingly close, and at times, so frustratingly distant.

Thus, if there is need to mention of another constant throughout my life, then faith and spirituality must be considered. As referenced earlier, my understanding of Christianity (and more so how it was to be practiced) was shaped by a series of trials. The first was related to the concept of hypocrisy. One of the most glaring issues that plagues the Church nowadays is the paradoxical nature in which its congregation interacts with one another. While the institution claims to be hospitable and welcoming to all who reside within it, there are several examples that allude to why it is anything but. Growing up, I greatly struggled with finding community in Church. I can remember the times in which my parents would drop me off outside of the doors of a Sunday youth program. Upon entering a room full of other similarly-aged children, I would assess what I could do or who I could talk to. I would start by kicking a soccer ball against the wall or would toss a basketball repeatedly into a nearby hoop. But in the end, there never happened to be any coincidental run-ins with another person who wanted to strike up conversation. And so, much of these instances saw me sitting alone, while other niche and selective groups would mingle and connect. Sure, I could make it through an hour and a half of a program until my parent's sermon had concluded, but it oftentimes felt as though I was praying the time away. Sundays were awkward and made me feel like a lonely outcast.

It wasn't as though I wasn't trying either. In anticipation of such Sundays, I would go through mental gymnastics to convince myself that attending Sunday school was worth it in the long run. After all, the program ought to have been valued for its primary purpose which was to educate youth about Christ, not to entertain trivial social quibbles. After a great deal of years, I found myself growing impartial, if not, apathetic towards the "youth group" scene. I had dug my feet into the earth and refused to admit myself into Sunday morning enrolment. Instead, I would obstinately sit beside Mom and Dad in the large auditorium, and listen to the pastor deliver his weekly message. My parents were clear about how they felt of my resolve, for they indicated that I wasn't "trying hard enough to put myself out there" to others. I imagine from their perspective that it was frustrating to have the one moment in the week away from their children be spoiled, but it also does not sit well with me knowing that they were unaware of my reasons for acting as such. We would sit in adjacent chairs during Sunday service, and a tone in the air suggested that we were further apart from one another in ways more than just proximal.

Fast forward to my freshman year of college; the year is 2014. Life for me had transitioned so quickly since graduating high school, and I had a one-track mind of how my expected 5-year timeline was to play out. In order to appease the satisfaction within me, I decided to calculate what I could do to acquire experience with youth before applying to the College of Education. I turned to my local church to solve two of my current problems. One, I would enrol as a youth leader to gain the required amount of volunteer hours (as well as acquire a professional reference) for my application. Two, there was a chance that in doing so I could establish fraternity with the other leaders and enjoy a community. While the first of those problems was solved, thankfully, the other followed a similar trajectory to that of my past. Other young adults came across as pretentious in their deeds. If conversation was had, much of it was shallow and cut short due to a seeming lack of interest. Once again, having read the room and realizing that others did not welcome me into their close-knit social circle(s), I turned attention to my responsibility at hand which was to mentor and care for a small group of middle aged youth.

When an opportunity arose for a young adult program to be housed through the church youth pastor's home, I swayed as to whether or not I should gamble on entering into another potential social deadlock. My pensiveness lasted for several weeks, months even, until I bit the bullet and drove to the planned location one weekday evening. The house was crammed with people, and my aversion to such scenes had already begun to stir from within my gut. I often reminded myself that God didn't make anything happen for those who simply waited for Him to act. Rather, it was the courageous and bold whom He granted deliverance. I would sit and chat with a stranger for minutes at a time, hoping that the sincerity and longing for conversation wouldn't be interpreted as desperation. But the conversations never lasted. People would begin to position themselves away from my direction and continue in earnest with someone else. As the weeks went by, I found myself sinking further and further internally. My initial curiosity for the group had turned to fatigue, which later turned into bitterness. Inevitably, I stopped attending. It was on the night of my final appearance that I shut the door to the house and made my way back to my parked car. I fumbled for the keys in my jacket pocket, unlocked the driver's-side door, and slid behind the steering wheel. After turning on the ignition, I placed both of my hands on 10-2 and closed my eyes. All I wanted to do in that moment was slam my skull against the wheel, maybe participate in a touch of masochism to make up for the emotional toil. It was in that moment that I genuinely asked God why He was making this all so impossible.

I heard a preacher once talk about the various ways in which God communicates with man. For some, God is audible like the voice of a man whose words carry with the wind. For others, He visits them in their dreams or provides them with visions about the future or what heaven will look like. But for many, they will note a resounding lack of theatrics. Supposedly, this final category makes up most Christians on Earth. By definition then, I would fall into this category.

Nothing would make me more aware of the presence of God than for Him to part the clouds in the sky with His hands and poke His head through the empty space and say "Levi, I'm real". However, I know that God is to be trusted by faith alone, and that He would never need to pander to a mere skeptic believer. It was this clarity of God's approach that made me realize that perhaps I had been anticipating a dramatic intervention for all of life's problems. There was also a large possibility that I was focused less on maintaining a personal relationship with the Lord, and more so on the things He could do to take me out of this stage one, earthly purgatory.

As I reflect on the many tribulations of my life, those mentioned in this book's recounting (as well as those that have not), a calming presence can still be detected in the background. This can be difficult to describe, for its composition takes no physical form. Consider the way that it feels to enter into a new situation, backed by the support of a close friend or person whom you trust. One would likely feel a semblance of comfort despite that other person not being physically there with them in the moment. I'm not quite sure why it took me so long to notice this presence. Perhaps I was too focused on "getting by" with little to no collateral. It could also be fair to assume that, for the longest time, I was simply living in the shadow of my parents' religion. I was being dragged along a path that was their journey, not mine.

It is with this realization that I began to compartmentalize my experiences and understandings of Christ. I began to ask the hard questions. When did (or have) I accept(ed) God as my personal Lord and Saviour? What is the role of a Christian in today's world? Have I actively pursued a life free of sin? Most importantly, what would it require for me to become subservient to the plans of a being whose knowledge of the universe is so vastly superior than my own? And with these questions gyrating from within the fabrics of my self-talk, I began to notice that familiar, surreal, and tranquil feeling weigh upon my shoulders once more. It was the Holy Spirit.

From then on, I began to consider the ethereal form of God and how it had remained beside me throughout my entire life. For example, given my already destitute relationship with the Church, it would have been easy to step away from religion altogether. Sure, I would have been urged to attend sermon every Sunday, like I had for years already at that point, but once I reached adulthood it would be within my full right to do so. But remarkably that didn't happen. Instead, I latched onto a hope that if I did not give up, something purposeful would result from it. And that is how I found Him.

In the hours of confusion, He is with me. In the hours of joyfulness, He is with me. Even in the hours of anguish, He is still with me. It's astounding, really, that God can take a broken down human and make him believe once more. Like a vessel guided by the beacon of a lighthouse, I remain indebted to God for never failing to guide me to shore. He's given me a renewed vitality towards things that are out of my control.

"Hi there, welcome to Tim Hortons. What can I get for you?" the voice digitized from the drive thru speaker. I leaned ever so slightly outside the driver's side window of my Saturn Ion coupe to respond.

"Yeah, I'll get two sausage and egg breakfast sandwiches in a combo with one medium double double and a medium hot chocolate". After confirming the order, I pulled up behind the other customers already present in the line-up. It was a Saturday, and I was headed to Tarah's condo to spend the day with her. Much of my thoughts preceding our day's planned events were overridden by a desire to do something meaningful for my (then) girlfriend. In between the stresses of post-secondary life, surprises didn't have to be extreme. Rather, it was the small, even mundane acts that spoke volumes. Tarah had always been so good at doing nice things for me, and perhaps I wanted to return the favour to even the slightest degree. As I approached the restaurant delivery window, I fumbled to get my wallet open to retrieve my debit card. With credit to the employee's efficiency, I juggled the tasks of passing them my card while having a bag of food virtually thrown all

the way into the adjacent passenger seat. As I placed the two drinks in each respective cupholder, I could hear the harsh chiming of the payment reader signalling some kind of error.

"I'm sorry," I apologized. "I might have to enter in the card and punch in my PIN," I suggested. Sometimes, the contactless service would be disrupted by a background technical error or perhaps the card was not placed on the machine long enough for the transaction to be registered. So, I tried once again, this time conducting my backup method. Once more, the machine cried its horrible tone, all the while displaying the following message in large capitalized font: "INSUFFICIENT FUNDS". Confused, I stared at the screen on the apparatus that lay in my hand. After a couple of seconds, the message disappeared and returned to its original suggestion of payment options and overall fee amount.

"There must be some kind of mistake," I commented. The cashier politely smiled and awaited my next move. I slipped my debit card back into its slot in my wallet and began to rifle through faded receipts and documents that had been stored within it for years. "There must be a twenty-dollar bill slumbering somewhere between these forgotten papers!" I assured myself. But alas, a miracle note never transpired. Instead, I clapped my hands together and placed them in-front of my mouth, almost as if to imprison a potential noise of disbelief that would overwhelm my urge to hold my greater emotions at bay.

"Sir?" the worker asked. Their voice was muffled, and a slight ringing like that of tinnitus could be felt permeating throughout my consciousness. I stuttered and stammered as my attention was slowly brought back towards the figure standing in the frame of the window.

"I can't... pay for this... I have no money," I muttered. The cashier did not respond. I then proceeded to grasp both hot drinks once more and passed them back through to the restaurant staff. The breakfast sandwiches, now likely cold due to the length of time I had spent

scouring for various payment solutions, were handed back as well. I then put my car into gear and solemnly made my way towards the nearby condo building.

Upon pulling into a visitor's parking stall, I took a moment to reconvene and reinforce my composure. What was I to tell Tarah? How bad would it look for her to be in a relationship with someone who had next to nothing in his bank account? Would this be enough for her to think that I may never live a day without being on the brink of bankruptcy?

***

For context, I was never irresponsible with my finances. In fact, I took great pride in being able to support several endeavours, given my circumstances of being a student and only being able to work part time on the weekends during the school year. For one, I was fortunate enough to own a vehicle that could get me both to and from various responsibilities. Secondly, the sheer weight of paying for university tuition (in full) every year was no easy feat. Mom and Dad were traditional in their understanding of my post-high school graduate life. If I was to stay at home, rent free, then I was to manage all of the other financial burdens I would experience. Given the quick turnaround between graduating high school and entering post-secondary, I felt compelled to take their offer. At least it would solve the challenge of securing room and board. Yet, as ideal as this contract sounded, it left out many of the blunt, crude conversations that were had amongst us three. Many of these conversations occurred when payments were to be made, but my clairvoyance on the matter spelled out impending danger. I wasn't looking for a handout per-se, but instead was desiring a compassionate response. Surely, given my folks' own troubles with money during their early years, they would be able to empathize? This was not often the case. It always came down to "what you can do more" to better yourself. This often related to suggestions, which honestly came forth in the form of decree or dogma. To them, I needed to work myself even harder than I already was. There was no room for self-prescribed grace.

I remember a time where my father picked me up from school one day. I was in middle school. And for reasons that I cannot recall, my siblings were notably absent. It must have been because I was at an after school basketball practice or was receiving extra math help from my teacher. Regardless, that return trip home had started out relatively peaceful. Dad asked me how my day was, to which I candidly responded with the expected distaste of a begrudged, hormonal teenager. I was thankful that he did not respond with provocation in this moment. For what eventually occurred during the car ride home would override any typical "coming-of-age" commentary.

As we turned the corner of the street that leads into the crescent of our neighbourhood, my Dad pulled over and switched off the ignition of his truck. Confused, I looked over to him and awaited some form of explanation.

"This may come as a surprise to you, and I don't expect you or your brothers to understand it fully yet, but I quit my job today". He was right, I didn't understand his decision in that moment. In fact, I was stunned. He went on to digress that our family would be fine, money-wise, despite him not securing a follow-up hire at another company in his career field. To that, I inquired as to how long it may take for him to do so. He didn't have a projected timeline, nor was it expected that he would have one. I wonder if in that moment whether or not my father was doing what I did in the kinds of situations where I approached him for monetary/life advice. What is it that he was wanting from me? I faintly remember providing him with some non-verbal assurance, mainly in the character of not freaking out or asking nonsensical questions. After ending our chat, we finished the leftover portion of our drive until we pulled the vehicle up and onto the concrete driveway of our family's property. In my mind, a seed of doubt concerning a new era of familial financial stability began to *root itself amongst the other concerns that had been planted long ago.*

***

After approximately ten minutes, I mustered up enough courage to exit my car and enter the condo building. The hallway was dimly lit by several yellow-bulbed lighting fixtures that were placed in-between tenant entry doorways. The fabric carpet that lined the floor was visibly worn to the point that one could tell which route received the most amount of foot traffic. As I passed each unit, the scent of a wide range of assorted foods could be noted. When I got to Tarah's door I paused and took a deep breath. I (think) had it all under control. The "knock, knock" of my knuckles rattled against the wood barrier. The door swung open and I was met with the wide-eyed fervour of my girlfriend. I smiled, a half-hearted smile, and just as I thought that I had made it through the initial moment of self-control, my lip began to quiver and my face contorted into an ugly assortment of shapes.

"What's wrong!?" Tarah asked as her initial joy evaporated and transformed into concern. But I could not vocalize in return. I practically fell into her figure, sobbing and lamenting my new predicament. It was not my proudest moment. I anticipated that my heightened state would need some time to simmer. Tarah ushered me into the unit and sat me down on the living room couch, all the while gingerly holding my hands and staring intently at my face. I later explained to her what had transpired earlier at the drive-thru. I told her of my intentions, and largely, my fears of what this development could have on our relationship. Needless to say, I spiralled into a pit of misery and she eventually pulled me out of it. This experience made me come to terms with a bona fide comorbidity to my childhood experiences, I developed a dread of money.

Things got better though, in this regard. Over time, Tarah and I worked together to find a solution towards limiting my negative responses towards financial stress. Much of this was possible because of her responsible awareness and understanding of banking and budgeting. I was her student, learning all sorts of things about finances that I had never heard of before. The term "interest rate" was a phrase that I had heard of, but never truly understood its significance or application, even though I had been locked into a horrendous bank loan plan needed to purchase my first vehicle. That decision was thanks to my parents. After making some changes to my practices, money began to trickle back into my account(s) and I stopped nervously checking my statements every day for fear of an account lock-out. Comparatively to the years before, I was in a time of bliss.

That being said, it would be a bold deception for me to state that money no longer holds me under its thumb. I still do not check my accounts regularly, not because of overflowing positive digits, but because of the "feelings" I experience when I see the numbers sprawled across a monitor screen. Even if the numbers appear healthy, they contain a weight to them that reflects a fragile, provisional existence. The reality is that the world functions around wealth. It has since the dawn of time, albeit in different mediums. But such standards can be thwarted by a repurposed take on what really matters in life.

Besides, how hard is it to make eggs and toast at home?

CHAPTER FIFTEEN

THE ROAD AHEAD

Forgiveness. It's the simplest thing to accept, yet the hardest to give. It takes various forms. At times, forgiveness looks like one person accepting the faults of another; and vice versa. Grace is bestowed as a parting gift and both groups move forward, leaving the hurt behind. Then there's the forgiveness of the self. One looks inward and enters into discussion with oneself, seeking understanding, acceptance, and a clean slate. And some people look above, to a higher power that can eradicate their tendencies to cling to intrusive thoughts. Prayers and petitions function as a request to have the Almighty cure the contagion that saps the healthy body. Whatever the shape or method, we all have a right to forgiveness.

However, in this dog-eat-dog, Darwinian world of ours, an

underlying societal code encourages the murder of the self and our abilities to forgive. It's seen as feeble; a reflection of a utopian ideal that is unfit for the model of 21st century lifestyle. Think of it! People cut corners in their workplace, socially, to undermine their peers and rise to the top of the food chain. Neighbours "compete" in a trivial contest of who can keep their lawn the most up-kept. Individuals choose a side on the political spectrum to align with in an effort to prove their commitment to particular ideologies and virtues. It is this sense of competition that drives many people's decisions to stand firm in their values. It is seen as better to die on the hill of broken relationships, so long as measurable success (by one's own evaluative criteria) is planted as a flag at the top of it. But what's missing from this way of living is the inherent magnetism that humans have had since their conception: the need for compatibility, dependence, and sympathy.

For so long I had been accustomed to keeping my thoughts inside. I told myself that my business had no business being heard by others. What more was such an act than but a perfect example of *The Boy Who Cried Wolf?* Looking back, it appears as straight masochism. My silence had been borne from both discomfort and a fear of the unknown. Alas, a turning point's trajectory changed the course of my life forever. Well, it may have very well been multiple instances rather than just a singular one. The constant in my life is good people. Genuine people who leaned in when others pushed away. I owe so much to them, and I pray that my words can suffice.

Now, despite the general improvement that I have experienced as of late, it would be ludicrous to fall under the illusion that things may never get difficult in the future. Life does not work that way. But gone are the days where I would remain silent and keep a cork on the bottle of my emotions. Emotions are meant to be felt, not dismissed. Moving forward, I vowed to be vocal and honest about where I was at and how I was feeling.

As a teacher, it was always interesting to determine how much of this practice could be applied to the realm of academia. Of course, a level of professionalism was to be upheld, but I never wanted to sell my soul (or identity) for the sake of a practice. So, I began to take baby-steps towards wearing my heart on my sleeve as an educator.

"How are you, Mr. S.?" a student would ask as they passed me by in the hallway.

"Good morning! You know, I'm feeling a little tired today. Nothing I can't get over though!" I would respond. It may not have been the expected response, but it was honest. I felt protective over the kids, and wanted to project to them a subliminal message that had the potential to mean far more than a history lesson.

During the final exam season of 2021-2022, I found myself adjudicating a group of grade twelve psychology students that were writing their end of semester exam. I assumed that most of them were eager to hand in their papers and get on with the rest of their lives. It had been a particularly enjoyable group of students to teach; the smaller class size was a result of it being an elective course option amongst other choices. We were able to discuss the curriculum in insightful and meaningful ways, as well as bond as individuals, as we talked about things not necessarily related to the scheduled lesson. I felt an increasing sense of self-worth as I taught them to learn about the human brain, its complexities, and how it can be man's biggest critic. Now that I mention it, maybe they thought I was crazy in my approach to the study.

I sat in my desk that afternoon marking exams, all the while keeping a close eye on the clock and the deadlines I needed to meet. As I scanned test answers, I flipped the page on one exam and paused at a response that appeared out of place. An arrow was drawn on the bottom right hand side of the page, indicating that something had been left on the backside of the paper. The following note read:

"SANTHA! Okay, so I finished writing my test and I just wanted to spend my extra time writing this note for you. I wanted to let you know that I appreciate you (a ton). You're a teacher that I won't forget because you impacted me a lot. I learned the importance of asking for help, being vulnerable, and being empathetic from you. You let your students genuinely be who they are, and you bring out the best in them. I love how you love your job and what you do because it helped me enjoy learning. Your eagerness to know more is contagious. :) You put your heart and soul into your work and making your classroom a safe space to just exist. You helped me get through this year with your empathy. You are so genuine about your responses to our struggles, and that's one of the biggest reasons why I'll miss you (but don't worry, I'll visit the school). I'll also miss your positive attitude towards learning, but I will carry it with me into college. What you have taught me about being kind and working hard will go with me through these next tough years. I'm really going to miss you and this class :(. You don't even know. BUT! When it's hard to say goodbye, it often means it was something very special. So, all that to say, thank you and I wish you all the best with the rest of your awesome career. :) -K"

Immediately, my eyes began to well up with emotion. Thankfully I was alone in the room at the time, for tears started to flow without restraint. For how critical I had been of myself in the past, I had other people in my life (young ones at that) telling me that what I was doing, who I was becoming, mattered to them. To them, I wasn't displaying the characteristics of a dark past. I was learning how to live with contagious vulnerability.

The truth of the matter is, I will never know what lies ahead. My twenties will undoubtedly come and go, leaving behind a significant chapter of my life that ended up being far more complex than originally anticipated. My treasured children will grow up, faster than I will want them to. First they will enter primary school and will then learn how to write their names within the lines of a piece of foolscap. They will also learn to make friends with others. I won't be physically there to assist them in these kinds of lessons. Something about that makes me nervous, and yet, I know that somehow it will all turn out just fine. It's a strange intuition.

Every new day will have its moments where decisions are to be made, with some feeling simple while others feel impossible. But what I do know is that I must have gone through the things I have, survived the things I was forced into, for some reason. If one thing is for certain, it is that with the right people in my life, and a modest level of self-esteem, maybe, just maybe, those decisions will be a little easier to make.

I don't know if I will ever be able to stare out at a field of canola like the way I did, all those years ago. Those glaring blots of yellow have undoubtedly stained a curious impression on me. The images of a blossoming prairie forever representing a symbolic period of my life where peace could be found in the simplest of things. What would life be without such moments?

So, to the person reading this, make sure that you do not let yourself falter as the result of something that was never in your control. It isn't fair to hold yourself accountable to a false standard that was created by the insecurities of trauma. Instead, be true to yourself and who you want to be. You deserve to craft a life that you want to live. You are you, and that person is meant to be heard and seen for some kind of beautiful purpose. Look after yourself.

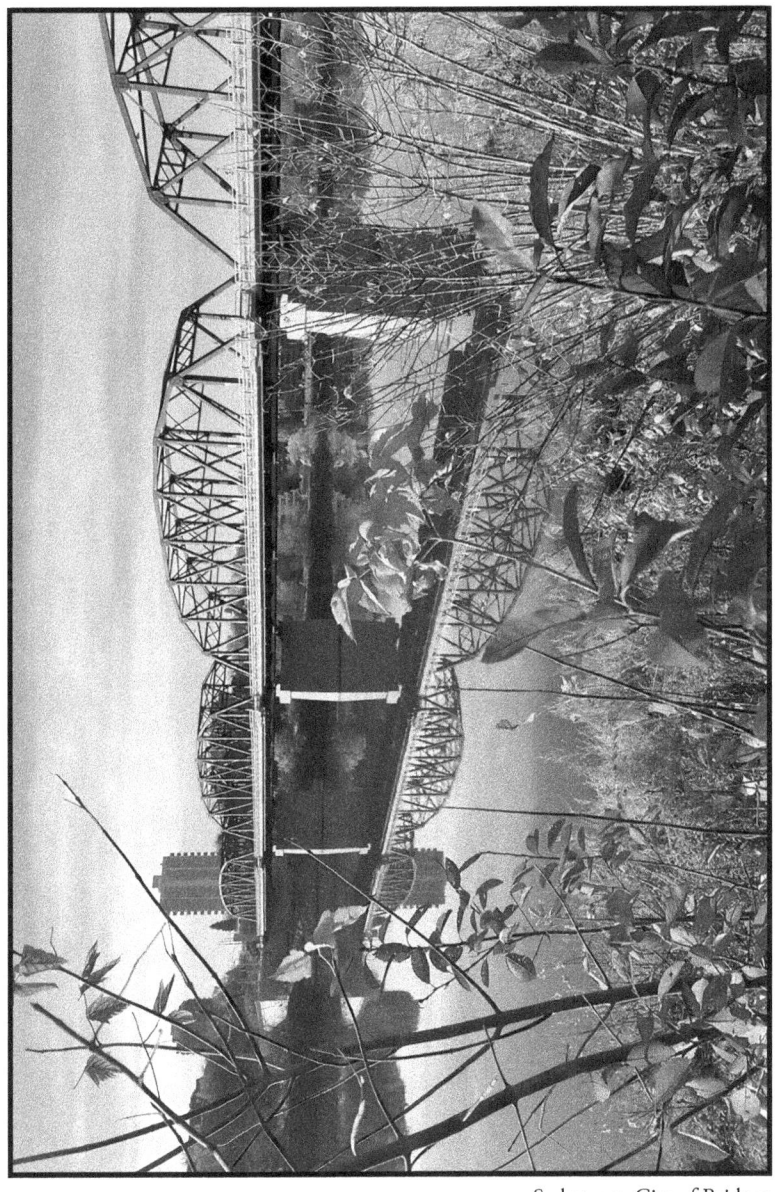

Saskatoon, City of Bridges

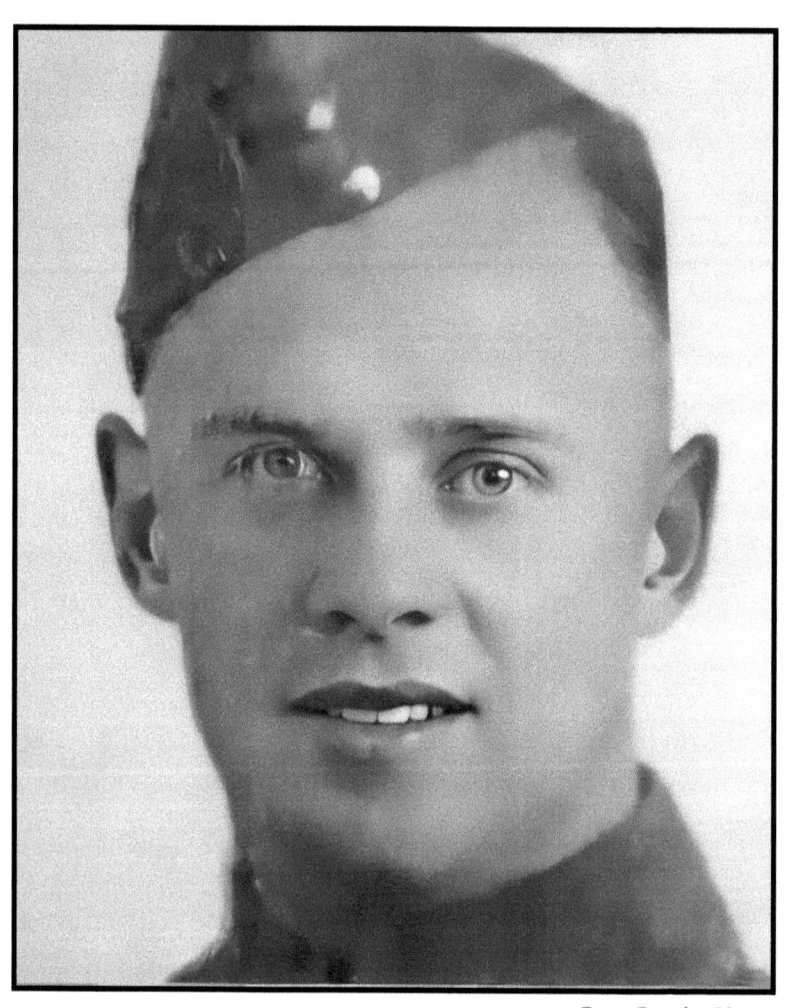

Great Grandpa Voysey

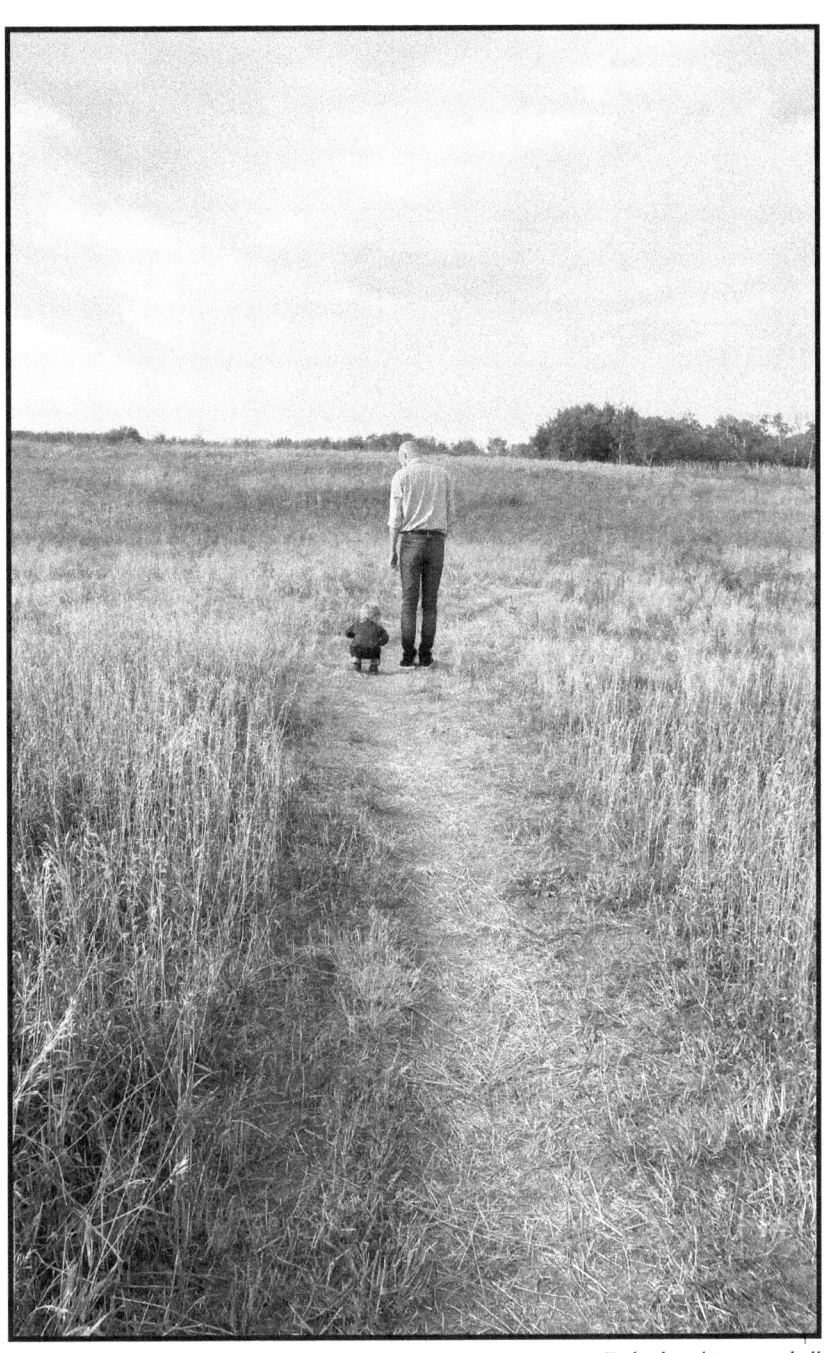

Fatherhood in a nutshell

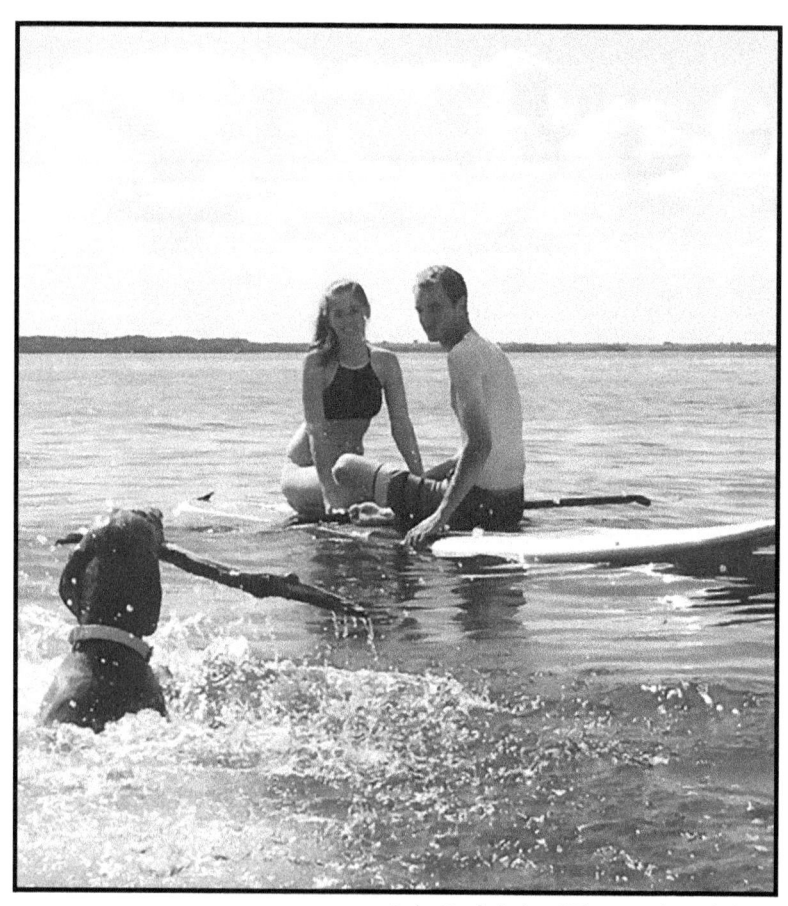

Lake Diefenbaker: Where my heart belongs

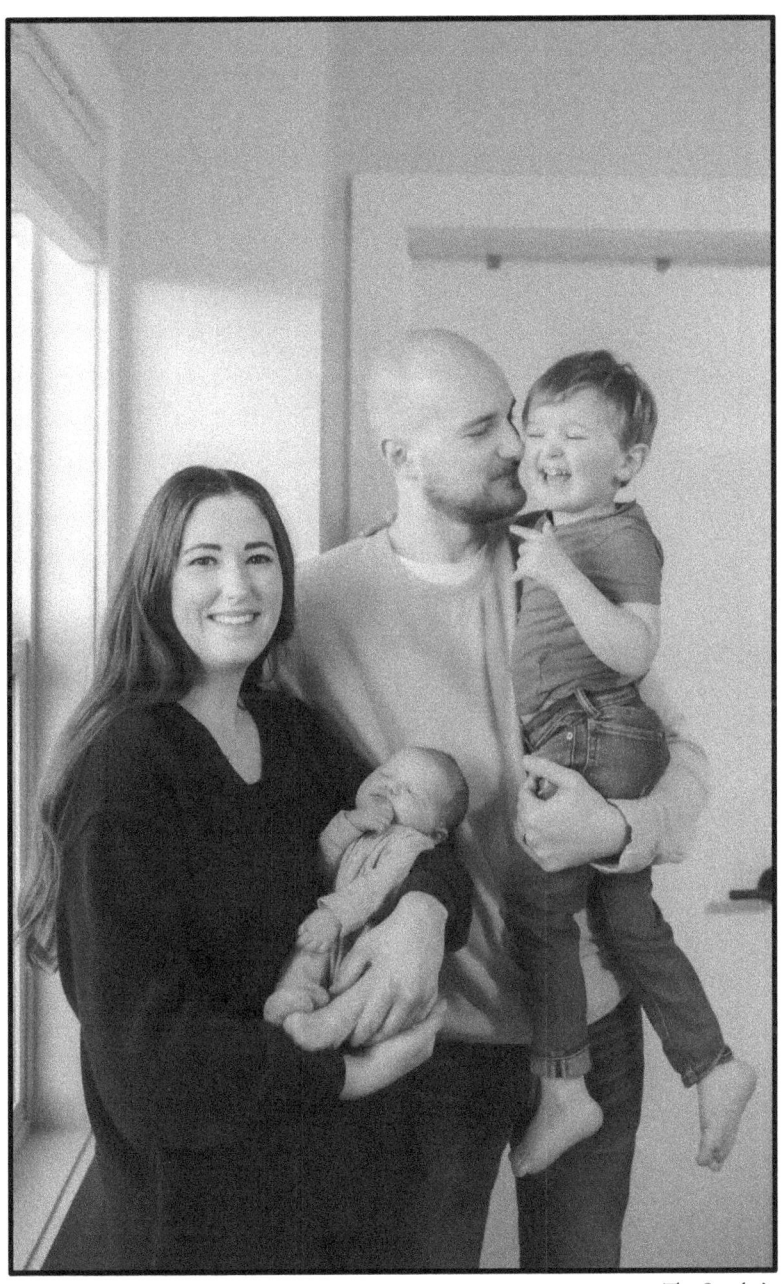

The Santha's

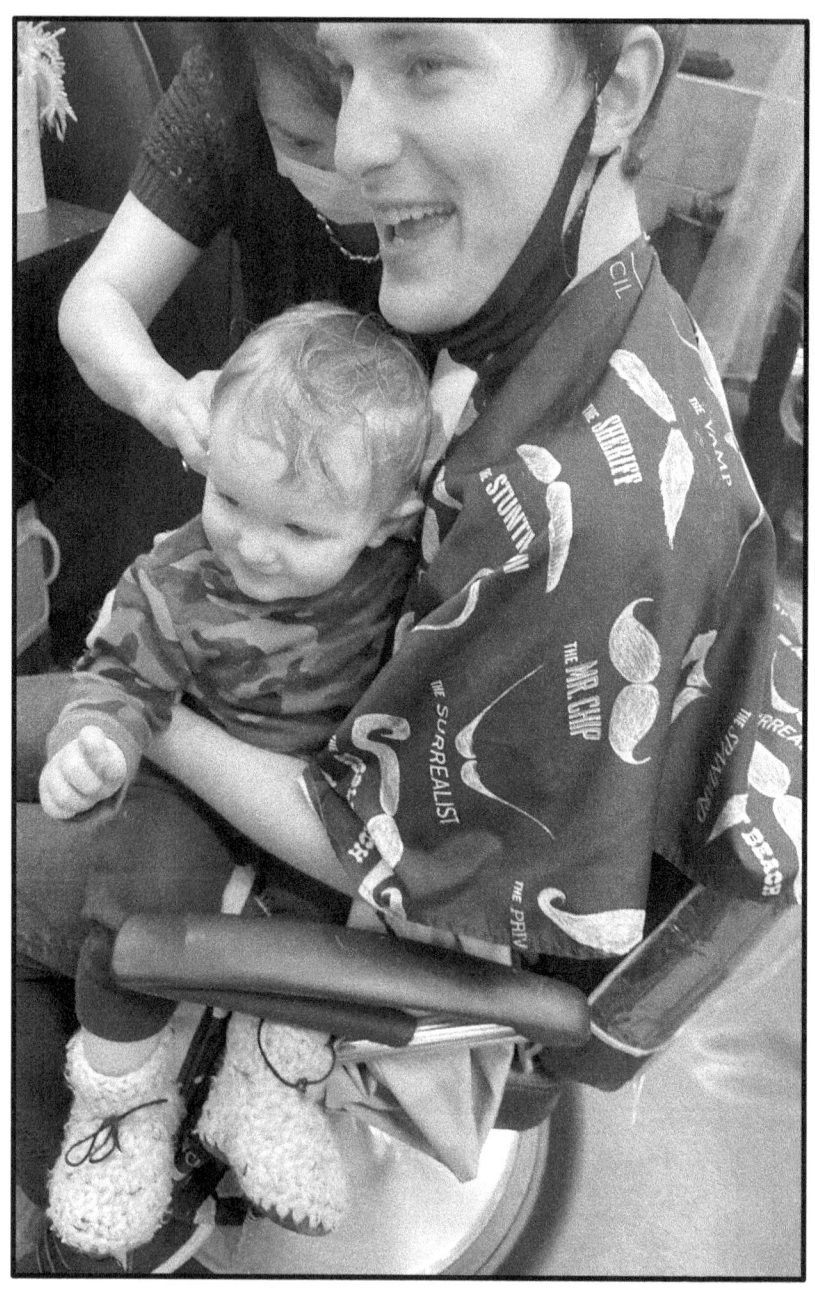

Life comes full circle

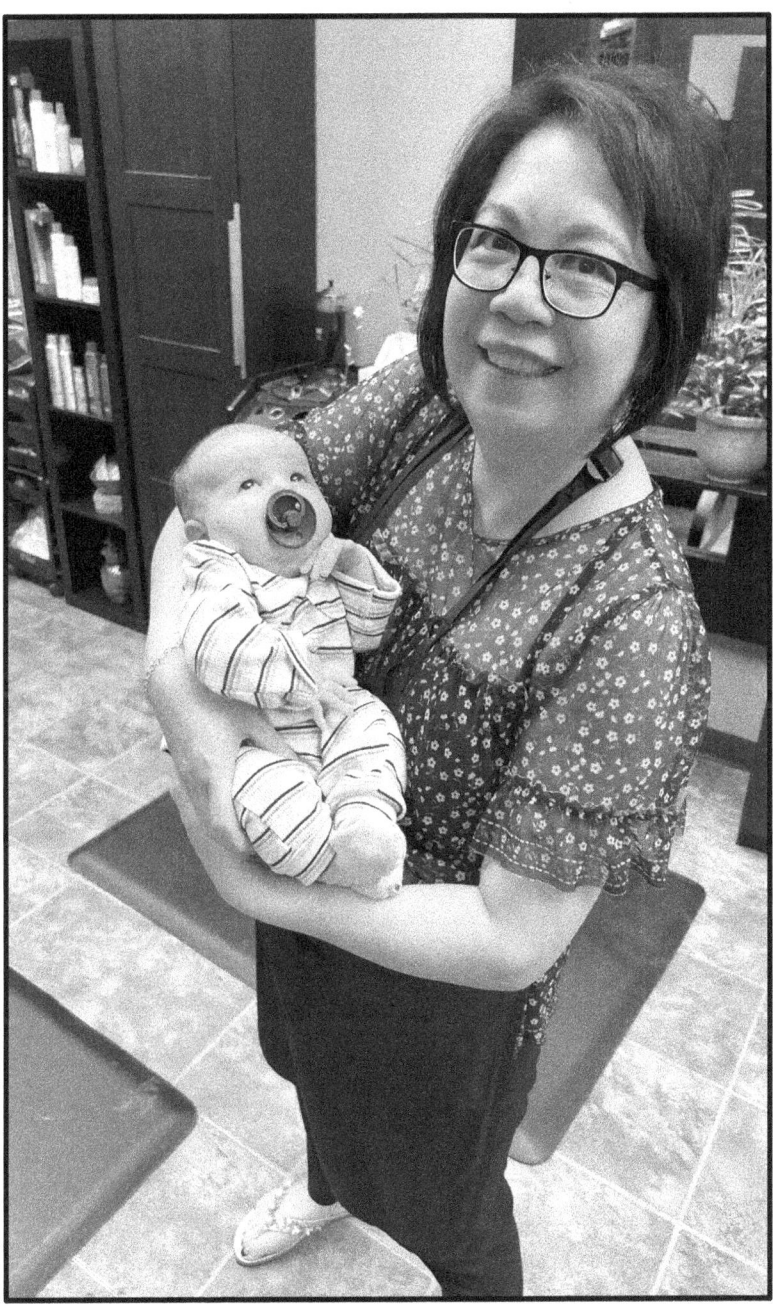

Julie: Hairdresser, therapist, adoptive mom

Santhaaaa

Psych. 30

okay, so I finished writing my test and I just wanted to spend my extra time writing this note for you. I wanted to let you know that I appreciate you (a ton). You're a teacher that I won't forget because you impacted me a lot. I learned the importance of asking for help, being vulnerable and being empathetic from you. You let your students actively be who they are and you bring out the best in them. I love how you love your job + what you do because it helped me enjoy learning. Your eagerness to know more is contagious. you put your heart and soul into your work and making your classroom a safe place to just exist. You helped me get through this year with your empathy. You are so genuine about your responses to our struggles and thats one of the biggest reasons I'll miss you :'(I'll also miss your positive attitude towards learning, but I will carry it with me into college. what you have taught me about being kind and working hard will go with me through these next tough years. I'm really gonna miss you and this class :' you don't even know. but! when it's hard to say goodbye it often means it was something very special. so all that to say thank you and I wish you all the best with the rest of your awesome career :'

"The student becomes the teacher"

ACKNOWLEDGMENTS

I would like to take a moment to acknowledge all of the people who made this book a reality.

A big thanks goes to Fay from Big Moose Publishing, whose unwavering communication and consistency allowed for this final product to appear exactly as intended.

Secondly, I would like to thank all of the individuals in my life who may or may not even be aware of the impact that they have had on me. This includes my close friends, family, and students both past and present.

Lastly, and most importantly, I would like to thank my wife, Tarah, for being an ever-present force whose devotion has kept me grounded and loved. If it were not for you, who is to say where I might be. I love you.

ABOUT THE AUTHOR

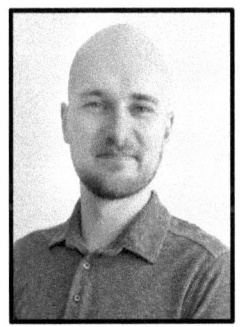

Levi Santha is a high school teacher who currently resides in Saskatoon, Saskatchewan.

Diagnosed with Generalized Anxiety Disorder (G.A.D.) in 2021, he began a personal journey to better understand the relationship between his mental health and his sensitive past. Seas of Yellow is his first work, and was created with the intent and purpose to help others realize that they are not alone with their thoughts or struggles.

Whether someone is looking to laugh, cry, or ponder over the intricacies of an anxiety-fuelled life, *Seas of Yellow* is sure to leave you thinking more about your own.